THE nephrotic syndrome

DISCUSSIONS IN PATIENT MANAGEMENT

Richard D. Wagoner, M.D.
Associate Professor of Medicine
Mayo Medical School
Consultant, Division of
Nephrology and Internal Medicine
Mayo Medical Clinic and Mayo Foundation
Rochester, Minnesota

Medical Examination Publishing Co., Inc.
an Excerpta Medica company

Wagoner, Richard D.
   The nephrotic syndrome--discussions in patient
management.

   Bibliography: p.
   Includes index
   1. Nephrotic syndrome--Treatment. I. Title. [DNLM:
1. Nephrotic syndrome--Therapy. WJ 340 W135d]
RC918.N43W33   616.6'1   81-11193
ISBN 0-87488-913-8   AACR2

Preface

Except for a few clinical conditions in which the nephrotic syndrome occurs, specific treatment is ineffective in producing a remission. The clinician, confronted with a newly recognized nephrotic patient, must by history, physical examination, and laboratory studies arrive at a working diagnosis before proposing a rational treatment program. Study of renal biopsy tissue usually is a necessary part of the evaluation, and close cooperation with a renal pathologist is important, as often no single finding is sufficient to make a proper diagnosis.

Whether or not a specific treatment is possible, one of the major tasks in the management of the nephrotic patient is to control edema formation, hypertension, and, later in the course, renal insufficiency. Frequently, this requires periodic reassessment because of the changing clinical situation. With sufficient background information, the clinician should be able to minimize morbidity in this condition and recognize potentially serious problems attendant upon the medical management of the patient. Hopefully, this book will provide a practical approach to the diagnosis and management of the patient with the nephrotic syndrome.

Acknowledgments

I wish to thank Mrs. Janice M. Graner, clinical dietitian, for her invaluable assistance; Dr. Marc A. Shampo for his editorial assistance; and Mrs. Judy K. Dugstad for typing the manuscript.

Continuing Medical Education Credits

As an organization accredited for Continuing Medical Education, Temple University School of Medicine has designated this continuing medical educational activity as meeting the criteria for 3 credit hours in Category I for educational materials for the Physician's Recognition Award of AMA, provided it has been completed according to instructions.

The purpose of this activity is to give information which the physician can apply to practice. By means of the self-assessment test the participant can evaluate the effectiveness of the educational experience.

Suggestions concerning the educational aspects of the program are encouraged and should be directed to:

Albert J. Finestone, M. D.
Associate Dean, Continuing Medical Education
Office for Continuing Medical Education
Temple University School of Medicine
3400 North Broad Street
Philadelphia, PA 19140

STATEMENT OF EDUCATIONAL OBJECTIVES

Following completion of this program, which is intended primarily for nephrologists, general internists and family practitioners, the reader will have a practical approach to the diagnosis and management of the patient with the nephrotic syndrome based upon the concepts stated in the Preface.

The participant will be able to test the effectiveness of this educational program by the completion of the self-assessment test.

Contents

notice

The editor(s) and/or author(s) and the publisher of this book
have made every effort to ensure that all therapeutic modalities that are recommended are in accordance with accepted
standards at the time of publication.

The drugs specified within this book may not have specific
approval by the Food and Drug Administration in regard to the
indications and dosages that are recommended by the editor(s)
and/or author(s). The manufacturer's package insert is the
best source of current prescribing information.

Chapter 1

INTRODUCTION

The nephrotic syndrome is often the predominant clinical manifestation of numerous diseases. Some of these diseases are primarily limited to the kidney, and others are systemic illnesses involving multiple organ systems. The commonly accepted minimal clinical criteria that are recognized as necessary for establishing a diagnosis of this syndrome include (1) a 24-hr urine protein excretion of 3.5 g or greater; (2) a serum albumin level of less than 3.0 g/dl; and (3) free lipids in the urine. Other frequently associated physical findings and laboratory abnormalities that may accompany this syndrome are peripheral edema, hypertension, hypercholesterolemia, hypertriglyceridemia, increased serum α_2-globulin level, and diminished serum γ-globulin level.

Most of the renal diseases that cause the nephrotic syndrome, with the possible exception of "nil lesion" nephrosis, also may occur without the syndrome. In the absence of nephrosis, these diseases usually produce some abnormalities of the urine, however. Remissions and exacerbations of the syndrome may occur either spontaneously during the natural course of a disease or as a response to treatment, and surprisingly, sometimes without an identifiable change in renal morphology. The syndrome thus is only the clinical expression of an underlying glomerular injury produced by any one of numerous possible diseases. Its presence should prompt the clinician to systematically search for an identifiable cause or , at the minimum, to provide the pathologist with kidney tissue for histologic classification of the renal morphology. With this information, decisions can be more competently made in regard to (1) planning specific treatment; (2) estimating renal function prognosis; and (3) providing information for the optimal treatment approach in the event that end-stage renal disease develops. Although only a few distinct primary renal lesions are amenable to treatment, numerous systemic diseases, with associated kidney involvement and this syndrome, are potentially treatable, often with resultant resolution of the nephrosis. Heavy proteinuria (> 3 g/24 hr) caused by exogenous toxins or sensitizing drugs also may either completely disappear or improve when the offending agent is eliminated.

Before planning an intelligent management program for the patient with the nephrotic syndrome, identification of the cause or classification of the renal morphology should be established. Frequently, this effort results only in a descriptive classification of the renal disease because most primary nephrologic disorders, with the exception of poststreptococcal glomerulonephritis, have no ostensibly identifiable cause. The same is true for many of the systemic diseases that result in renal damage. Interestingly, when other diagnostic efforts have failed, the initial recognition of one of these systemic diseases finally may be made only after examination of renal tissue. Although the syndrome infrequently is due to exogenously administered toxins such as heavy metals, some medications, and certain infections, identification of any of these potential causes is crucial because successful resolution can be expected with appropriate management.

Table 1 lists the classification of primary renal diseases and systemic diseases known to be associated with the nephrotic syndrome. Other lesser categories include infections, malignancies, and exogenously administered toxins. The five broad categories offer the clinician direction for a systematic approach in pertinent history taking, physical examination, and laboratory evaluation of the nephrotic patient. The list can facilitate an awareness of an already established disease as the probable cause of this syndrome when heavy proteinuria develops later in its course—for example, in diabetes mellitus, systemic lupus erythematosus, or lymphoma. In addition, the list may be helpful in alerting the clinician to suspect the presence of the nephrotic syndrome in certain clinical settings when it is not overtly apparent. Finally, this classification provides a reference for those diseases in which, during their natural course, the nephrotic syndrome might be expected to eventually develop.

While the initial efforts are necessarily focused on determining the cause of the syndrome or the renal morphologic changes accompanying it, it is also necessary for the clinician to be familiar with the acute and chronic management of several concurrent clinical problems: (1) edema formation; (2) hypertension; (3) renal insufficiency; and (4) end-stage renal disease.

Table 1   Etiologic and Renal Morphologic Classification of the Nephrotic Syndrome

---

A. Primary renal diseases
1. Idiopathic membranous glomerulopathy
2. Membranoproliferative glomerulonephritis
3. Idiopathic proliferative glomerulonephritis
4. Focal sclerosing glomerulopathy
5. "Nil lesion"
6. IgG-IgA nephropathy
7. Idiopathic rapidly progressive glomerulonephritis
8. Congenital nephrosis
9. Hereditary nephrosis

B. Associated systemic diseases
1. Diabetes mellitus
2. Amyloidosis—primary and secondary
3. Systemic lupus erythematosus
4. Goodpasture's syndrome
5. Fabry's disease
6. Sickle cell disease
7. Essential mixed cryoglobulinemia
8. Waldenstroem's macroglobulinemia
9. Vasculitides
   Periarteritis nodosa
   Wegener's granulomatosis
   Schoenlein-Henoch syndrome
   Nonspecific

C. Neoplasia
1. Lymphoproliferative disease
2. Solid tumors —colon, lung, pancreas, stomach

D. Infections
1. Acute poststreptococcal glomerulonephritis
2. Bacterial endocarditis
3. Infected atrioventricular shunt
4. Syphilis, secondary
5. Parasitic—malaria, filariasis, schistosomiasis, trypanosomiasis

E. Exogenous toxins—noninfectious
1. D-Penicillamine
2. Trimethadione
3. Gold
4. Mercury
5. Bismuth
6. Heroin (with bacteremia)
7. Nonsteroidal anti-inflammatory agents
8. Miscellaneous

Chapter 2

CLINICAL FEATURES

<u>Physical Findings</u>

Most mephrotic patients, whether the condition is well controlled or not, have edema. The mechanism for the formation
of this edema is depicted in Fig. 1. After glomerular damage
(which may be due to one of multiple mechanisms), serum albumin levels are reduced, primarily because of the large losses of urinary protein filtered through the altered glomerular

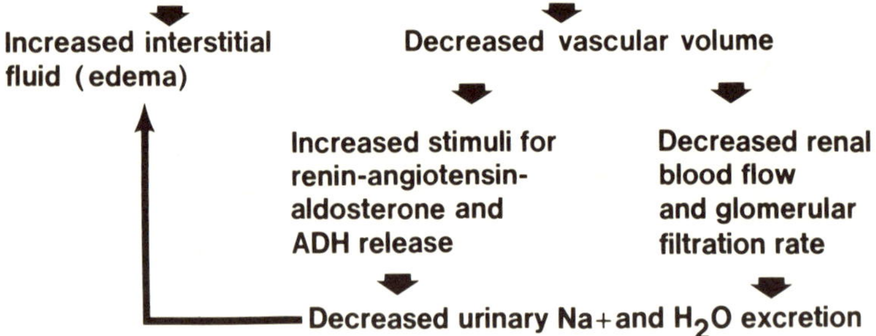

Fig. 1   Mechanism of edema formation in the nephrotic
syndrome.

basement membrane, exceeding the body's protein-synthesizing capacity. There is also probably increased renal tubular catabolism of the filtered urine protein because measured urinary loss alone cannot account for the total reduction in serum albumin level. [The resultant decreased plasma oncotic pressure initiates three mechanisms that contribute to the formation and persistence of edema: (1) loss of intravascular fluid into interstitial tissue; (2) stimulation of the renin-angiotension-aldosterone system and release of antidiuretic hormone from this decreased vascular volume; and (3) reduction in both renal plasma flow and glomerular filtration.] The second and third mechanisms are normal physiologic responses to the first.

The second and third mechanisms are also physiologic attempts to restore vascular volume by decreasing urinary sodium and water excretion. However, [because this retained sodium and water cannot be effectively contained in the vascular space (due to decreased plasma oncotic pressure), no overriding mechanism exists which can turn off excess renin stimulation or antidiuretic hormone release and improve glomerular filtration.] Consequently, the stimuli for edema accumulation persist.

A very small percentage of nephrotic patients, usually young adults, may remain virtually edema-free, even without the aid of diuretics and a sodium-restricted diet. These patients, because their protein intake is generous and their urinary protein excretion is relatively low, can maintain near-normal levels of serum albumin. Generally, the nephrotic patient with persisting heavy proteinuria who becomes edema-free, however, has been overly diuresed by vigorous attempts at extracellular fluid control; physical signs of hypovolemia, such as poor tissue turgor, dry mucous membranes, and orthostatic hypotension in particular, are readily apparent.

Edema formation in the lower extremities is characteristically symmetrical. When it is not, other medical conditions should be considered, such as unilateral deep venous insufficiency and acute sural or ileofemoral thrombophlebitis. (Nephrotic patients have coagulation abnormalities that make them particularly susceptible to venous-thrombosing tendency.[1]) Other considerations causative of asymmetrical edema include malignancies with unilateral lymphatic or venous obstruction and disparate use of the extremities secondary to diseases of the nervous system or to arthritic diseases.

Ascites is common. When it is excessive, however, and out of proportion to the edema formation in the lower extremities, its presence is suggestive of intraabdominal metastatic malignancy or obstruction of the vena cava secondary to tumor or thrombosis. Facial edema, worse in the morning and often asymmetrical if the patient sleeps on his side, diminishes during the day and seldom is a cosmetic problem, except in young children whose general edema is frequently more difficult to manage. Usually, the lower the level of serum albumin, the greater the tendency toward edema formation. Patients with serum albumin levels less than 1.5 g/dl invariably present difficult problems in the management of their extracellular fluid excess.

Pleural effusions occur frequently, most often bilaterally, increasing or regressing together with the status of control of peripheral edema. Effusions, especially unilateral and associated with pleuritic pain, are more often the result of pulmonary emboli, an occasional complication of the nephrotic syndrome. At times, these pleural effusions are a source of significant dyspnea and require thoracentesis for symptomatic relief.

Distension of the neck veins more than normal in nephrotic patients is rarely seen in the absence of cardiac decompensation, chronic obstructive lung disease, or obstruction of the superior vena cava. Similarly, pulmonary rales, wheezing, and laryngeal edema (enough to cause respiratory distress) are rarely caused by the nephrotic state. Edema of the genitalia, even though uncomfortable, is not a potential cause of obstructive uropathy.

Fortunately, the distended, edematous skin of nephrotic patients is not unusually sensitive to trauma. The skin heals slowly from injury (sometimes iatrogenic), however; surgical incisions in edematous areas may separate shortly after closure and heal indolently. Cellulitis develops more commonly in edematous limbs, often spreading very rapidly if not recognized and treated early.

Hypertension is a variable occurrence in the nephrotic syndrome. Uncommon in untreated patients with "nil lesion" nephrosis, it is frequent in acute poststreptococcal glomerulonephritis and is not unusual in many other renal diseases. If treatment of the nephrotic syndrome with corticosteroids is required, invariably the problem of hypertension emerges or pre-existing blood pressure elevation is exaggerated. In this group

of hypertensive nephrotic patients, resolution of heavy proteinuria may not necessarily be accompanied by a return to normo-
tension if the underlying renal lesion persists and particluarly
if renal function is deteriorating.

Laboratory Findings

Nephrotic patients have a number of laboratory test abnormalities that readily help in diagnosis. Unfortunately, these are
frequently nonspecific, providing little information about the
nature of the underlying renal disease. On occasion, however,
by their presence or absence, certain laboratory abnormalities
are predictable indicators of a specific disease process. (More
definitive laboratory tests beyond the basic nephrotic workup
are reviewed in Chap. 3, "Principles of Evaluation.") The following laboratory abnormalities are common to all nephrotic
patients.

Urinalysis

A concentrated urine specimen, preferably the first morning
fasting sample, when tested by the dipstick method, qualitatively shows proteinuria (grade 4 or 1,000 mg/dl) with di-
lute specimens, grade 3 (300 mg/dl) readings are not rare, but
values less than this are observed only during a massive diuretic state. Because the dipstick test does not reveal the presence of Bence Jones protein, some laboratories routinely
screen for proteinuria with the sulfasalicylic acid or heat and
acetic acid test, which will also detect isolated urinary light-
chain proteins.

By definition, urine of the nephrotic patient contains free
lipids that are readily detectable by microscopic examination of
the sediment from a centrifuged specimen (Fig. 2). These lipids also exist as oval fat bodies (Fig. 3, top left) and cast-
containing lipids or fatty casts (Fig. 3 top right). Sediment abnormalities, such as fats from specimen contamination, have
an appearance similar to these lipids, and therefore, the sediment also should be examined microscopically with polarized
light (Fig. 3, middle left and right and bottom left). Lipid material in the urine is doubly refractile because of its cholesterol
content, whereas contaminants do not have this characteristic.
Also similar in appearance to fatty casts are red cell casts; differentiation between the two types is not difficult though—material in fatty casts is of variable size, in contrast to that in
red cell casts; and polarized light readily reveals the doubly
refractile bodies characteristic of lipid casts. These lipids

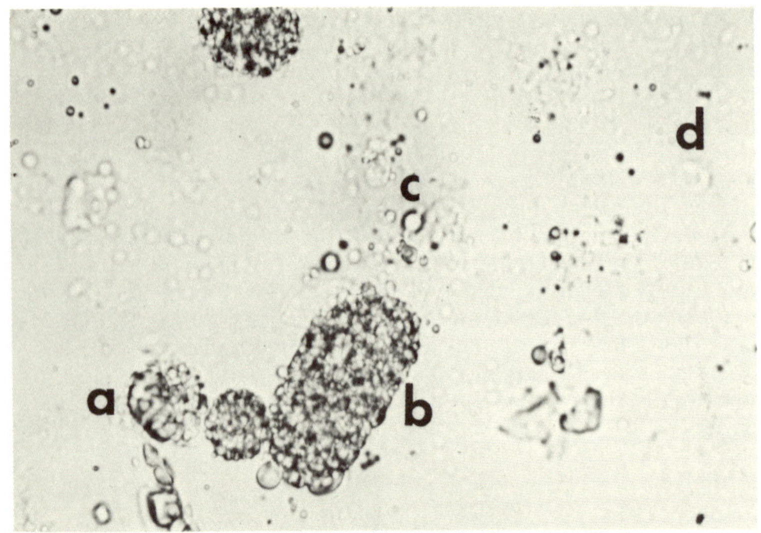

Fig. 2 High-power light microscopy shows size comparisons of urine sediment: (a) oval fat body; (b) fatty cast; (c) free lipids, (d) red cell.

abnormalities in urine sediment, however, are not unique to the nephrotic syndrome, as they are also present in urine that has lesser degrees of proteinuria. In contrast, heavy proteinuria can be present on rare occasions without lipids in the urine. This finding is highly suggestive of isolated light-chain proteinuria secondary to a disorder such as multiple myeloma in which hypoalbuminemia may not be an associated feature (unless complicated by renal amyloidosis).

Microscopic hematuria and urinary casts of types other than fatty casts are variable findings. The presence or absence of red blood cells, hemoglobin casts, and red blood cell casts can have significance in the preliminary differential diagnosis of the nephrotic renal disorder and will be discussed in Chap. 3, "Principles of Evaluation."

Much has been written about the diagnostic importance of the relative amounts of various-sized proteins in the urine of patients with the nephrotic syndrome, that is, the usefulness of determining "selective" versus "nonselective" proteinuria.[2] "Selective proteinuria" is characterized by a high percentage of

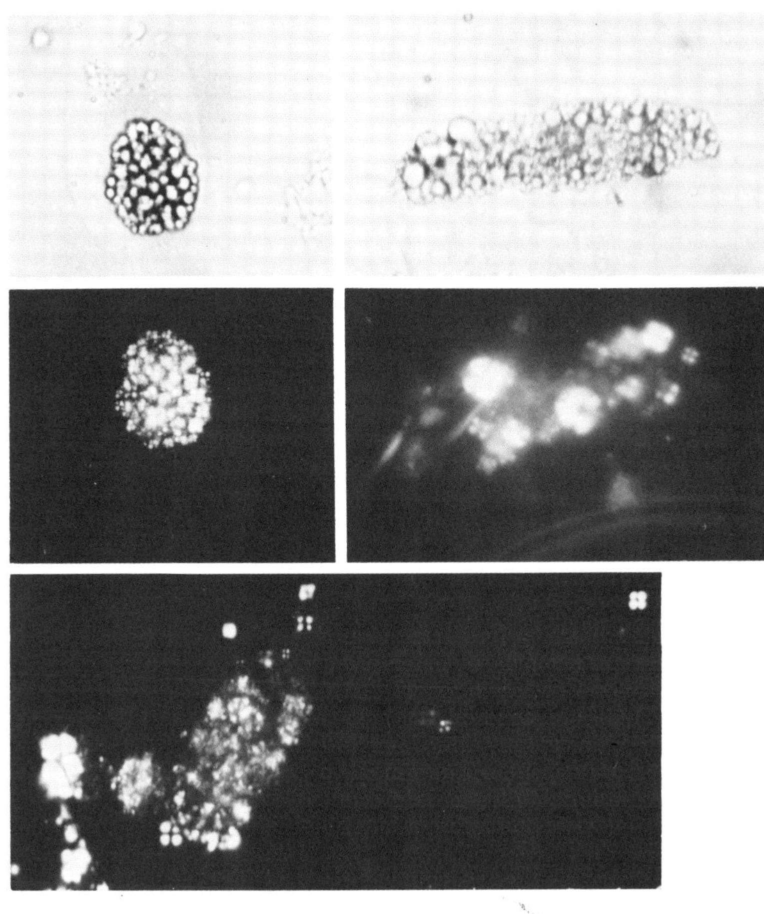

Fig. 3 Urine sediment: (top left) oval fat body under high-power light microscopy; (top right) fatty cast under high-power light microscopy; (middle left) oval fat body under high-power polarized light; (middle right) fatty cast under high-power polarized light; (bottom left) free lipids (maltese crosses) under high-power polarized light.

low-molecular-weight proteins, predominantly albumin, and implies a potentially favorable response to treatment. Nonavailability of techniques in most laboratories for performing this study and the overlap between the two categories of protein selectivity in clinical disorders have diminished its usefulness, however, as a practical laboratory test.

Serum Protein Abnormalities

Common abnormalities of serum proteins demonstrable on paper electrophoresis consist of a variable reduction in the serum albumin fraction to levels sometimes lower than 1.0 mg/dl, a small increase in the α_2 and β-globulin fractions and a γ-globulin fraction that is usually less than normal (Fig. 4). When the γ-globulin fraction is elevated, the possibilities of such clinical disorders as the dysproteinemias or systemic lupus erythematosus should be considered. The major factors

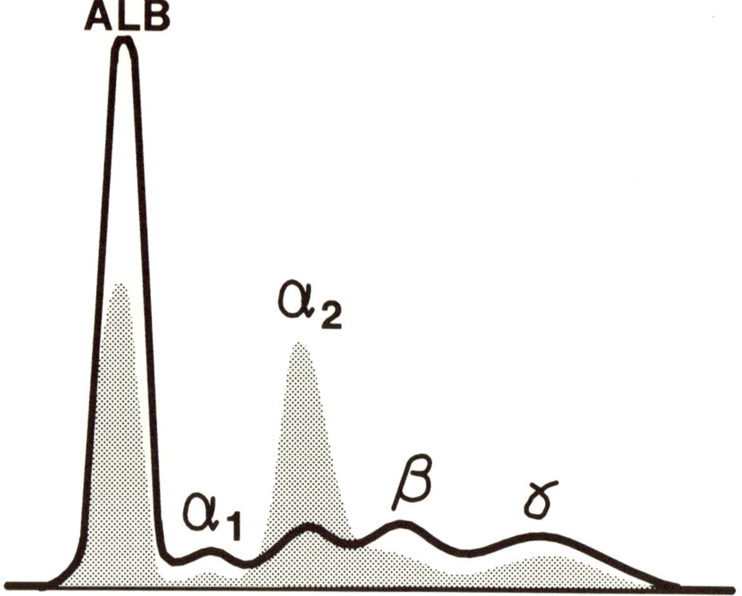

Fig. 4 Serum protein electrophoretic profile in nephrotic syndrome.

influencing these serum protein changes are (1) excessive loss
of protein in the urine; (2) increased catabolism of protein by
the renal tubules; (3) decreased synthesis of protein secondary
to dietary alterations; and (4) the theoretical influence of decreased plasma oncotic pressure on protein synthesis. The
mechanisms by which these factors exert their influence on
serum proteins, other than excessive urine protein loss, however, have not as yet been clearly delineated. Infrequently, the
patient with a heavy intake of dietary protein may maintain the
serum albumin level in near-normal concentrations despite
heavy proteinuria, but usually the abnormalities of other serum
protein fractions previously mentioned exist.

Electrolyte Abnormalities

Nephrosis itself seldom is responsible for clinically significant
changes in serum electrolytes. Levels of serum calcium are
consistently reduced, predominantly a secondary effect of diminished protein binding from hypoalbuminemia. Some evidence indicates that the ionized serum calcium fraction is also
reduced and that intestinal calcium absorption is impaired.[3]

Serum sodium concentration is normal unless influenced by
vigorous diuretic measures, and then the concentration may be
either elevated or decreased, depending on the diuretic program used. Spuriously low levels of serum sodium can be seen
with greatly elevated levels of serum cholesterol, because the
usual method of sodium determination measures the serum
concentration only and not the plasma water concentration. In
this instance, a greater-than-normal percentage of the serum
volume is composed of lipids, which displace plasma water.

Levels of serum potassium and uric acid, when abnormal,
are almost always diuretic-related or influenced by the level of
renal function. The combination of elevated levels of serum
uric acid and serum potassium frequently occurs with advanced
renal insufficiency, while an elevated serum uric acid level
and a decreased serum potassium level are suggestive of the
influence of the diuretic agent.

Lipid Abnormalities

Levels of serum cholesterol and triglycerides are usually increased and have an inverse relationship to the level of serum
albumin. The most frequent class of lipid abnormality is either
a type II or IIB.[4] Unexplained as yet are the mechanisms that
alter the serum lipid levels. Increased hepatic synthesis of

low-density lipoproteins and very low-density lipoproteins, as well as excessive lipid mobilization from body stores, have been postulated as mechanisms.[5] The influence of hypoalbuminemia may be a factor also, as a cholesterol-lowering effect has been noted experimentally when low plasma oncotic pressure is increased.[6]

Chapter 3

PRINCIPLES OF EVALUATION

A combination of accurate historical information, appropriate
laboratory data, and expert examination of renal tissue reviewed by clinician and pathologist in concert is the most effective
method of reaching an accurate diagnosis of the clinical problem responsible for the nephrotic syndrome. Evaluation of the
patient frequently begins with assessment of an edematous state
that has developed insidiously during a period of days to several
weeks. Typically in the adult, there is a gradual and progressive gain of weight, followed by the appearance of edema,
usually in the lower extremities first. On direct questioning,
patients often affirm a recognized change in their urine, which
has become foamy in appearance. The presence of heavy proteinuria on a routine urinalysis should initiate a history carefully taken with special regard to several points of information.
This historical information is particularly important for two
reasons. First, positive elements of the history help determine which of many laboratory tests will be most productive in
defining a cause or in clarifying the differential diagnosis of a
renal morphologic lesion. Second, a number of causes such as
drugs, infections, or tumors frequently are associated with a
common but nonspecific renal morphologic change.

History

Documentation of previous normal findings on urinalysis aids
in estimating when the renal disease began. However, many of
the diseases listed in Table 1 (Chap. 1) can be preceded by long
periods of asymptomatic proteinuria. The patient with long-
standing diabetes mellitus and minimal proteinuria who subsequently becomes nephrotic is a common example of this. If a
general estimate of when the nephrotic syndrome began is possible, patients should be queried as to a temporally related
upper respiratory or dermal infection or the passage of abnor-
mally colored urine (experienced, for example, in acute

poststreptococcal glomerulonephritis). Recurrent gross, painless hematuria closely associated with upper respiratory infections or flulike illnesses is commonly observed in IgG-IgA nephropathy.[7] (Heavy proteinuria is not a frequent feature of this particular renal lesion, but when present, it is an ominous prognostic sign.) A history of painless gross hematuria is also not uncommon with the morphologic lesion membranoproliferative glomerulonephritis.[8]

Specific questions regarding the use of certain medications should be asked, because patients may not always volunteer this information or may not consider some drugs as medication. This is well exemplified by the nephrotic patient who has used ammoniated mercury for many years as a treatment for psoriasis but does not consider topical ointments as medication. Specific inquiry about the psoriasis treatment may lead to the correct etiologic diagnosis (that is, mercury).[9] Among the few recognized drugs known to cause nephrosis, perhaps D-penicillamine[10] used in the treatment of patients with Wilson's disease, patients who are cystine stone formers, and patients with rheumatoid arthritis is most often implicated. Recently, nonsteroidal anti-inflammatory drugs[11] and the new antihypertensive agent captopril also have been reported as causing nephrosis.[12]

Persisting chronic infections, notably tuberculosis or osteomyelitis, and the disease Mediterranean fever[13] are the most frequent causes of secondary amyloidosis with the nephrotic syndrome. Pronounced fatigue, objective muscle weakness, and unexplained cardiac decompensation in a nephrotic patient are suggestive of primary amyloidosis.[14] When patients experience flank pain, sometimes with gross hematuria, the diagnosis of membranous glomerulopathy with renal vein thrombosis should be suspected. Symptoms compatible with lower-extremity thrombophlebitis or pulmonary emboli or both are similarly important clues to this diagnosis.

A form of hereditary nephritis is associated, on rare occasion, with nephrosis.[15] A strong family history of premature death from renal disease and members with hearing and visual impairment developing at an early age typify this genetically transmitted disorder (Alport's syndrome).

The symptom complex of varying combinations of arthralgias, fever, pleuropericardial pain, seizures, skin rash, and Raynaud's phenomenon when associated with nephrosis is suggestive of the possibility of systemic erythematosus, a nonspecific vasculitis, or primary mixed cryoglobulinemia.[16]

Hemoptysis in the absence of pleuritic pain might be the initial manifestation of Goodpasture's syndrome or one of the vasculitides. When this symptom accompanies nephrosis, it is not uncommon that the differentiation must await histologic examination of renal, respiratory mucosal, or other body tissue.

Purpuric skin lesions are suggestive of such diagnoses as the vasculitides, essential mixed cryoglobulinemia, and Schoenlein-Henoch disease.[17]

Patients with sickle cell disease who manifest heavy proteinuria are most likely to have renal involvement secondary to their red cell defect.[18]

Many of the systemic diseases previously mentioned are associated with fevers. Also, bacterial endocarditis may present with fever and heavy proteinuria, mimicking these other disorders.[19]

Basic Laboratory Data

Certain fundamental laboratory examinations are recommended in the evaluation of the patient with a newly recognized nephrotic syndrome. These studies, in addition to providing preliminary information for diagnostic help, are useful in planning immediate and future management programs. Suggested tests included in the basic blood studies are the following: (1) hemoglobin, leukocyte, and platelet counts; (2) serum creatinine, sodium, potassium, uric acid, and plasma glucose; (3) serum protein electrophoresis; (4) antistreptolysin O titer; (5) serum whole complement; (6) antinuclear antibody titer; and (7) erythrocyte sedimentation rate.

Urine studies should include routine urinalysis with microscopic sediment examination and 24-hr urine protein quantitation, preferably with a protein electrophoresis determination.

Sophisticated assessment of renal function with tests such as the creatinine clearance, radioactive[125I] iothalamate, and inulin and p-aminophippuric acid clearance studies can be misleading and should be interpreted with caution in nephrotic patients. Changes in vascular volume from hypoalbuminemia, for example, may introduce a prerenal variable that is difficult to assess. The timed urine collection necessary for these determinations also may be a source of error because of low urine flow rates.

Roentgenographic Data

Roentgenographic studies should include, as a minimum, a kidney-ureter-bladder roentgenogram without contrast medium for determination of renal size and for possible use in kidney localization at the time of percutaneous renal biopsy. Excretory urography should be considered since it provides more information than a plain renal area roentgenogram in the evaluation of the collecting system and in outlining abnormal renal masses (if renal function is not so severely impaired that little contrast medium is excreted). Some precaution is necessary when deciding on urography, however. Contrast-medium-induced acute renal failure is now recognized as a significant potential hazard. This is particularly of concern in diabetic patients and possibly in nondiabetic patients with renal function less than 50% of normal.[20,21] Unless indications other than nephrosis exist, urography should not be used as part of the evaluation of a diabetic or nondiabetic patient with advanced renal failure. Also in this clinical setting, the use of contrast medium during a fluoroscopically assisted renal biopsy procedure is potentially hazardous. Excretory urography sometimes is informative, however, in a very positive way, particularly in patients who have histories of thromboembolic incidents or flank pain and gross hematuria. Roentgenographic features that are highly suggestive of renal vein thrombosis or inferior vena cava thrombosis or both include unilaterally or bilaterally enlarged kidneys, narrowed and elongated infundibula, delayed appearance of contrast medium, extrinsic focal compression of the renal pelvis and ureters, and a pear-shaped bladder appearance (Fig. 5); the last two mentioned features are secondary to enlarged venous collateral channels. The roentgenographic procedures used for definitive diagnosis of renal vein thrombosis will be discussed later. Roentgenographic abnormalities of the chest, such as infiltrates from pulmonary emboli or an enlarged azygos vein secondary to collateral venous return after thrombosis of the inferior vena cava, also should be considered clues to renal vein thrombosis.

Renal Biopsy

Examination of renal tissue is an integral part in the evaluation of the nephrotic patient. The technique of percutaneous renal biopsy has been well established and is an acceptable procedure for obtaining tissue. In the hands of experienced personnel, renal tissue adequate for examination is obtained by the percutaneous technique approximately 95% of the time. A complication rate of about 7% has been noted in several large series.[22]

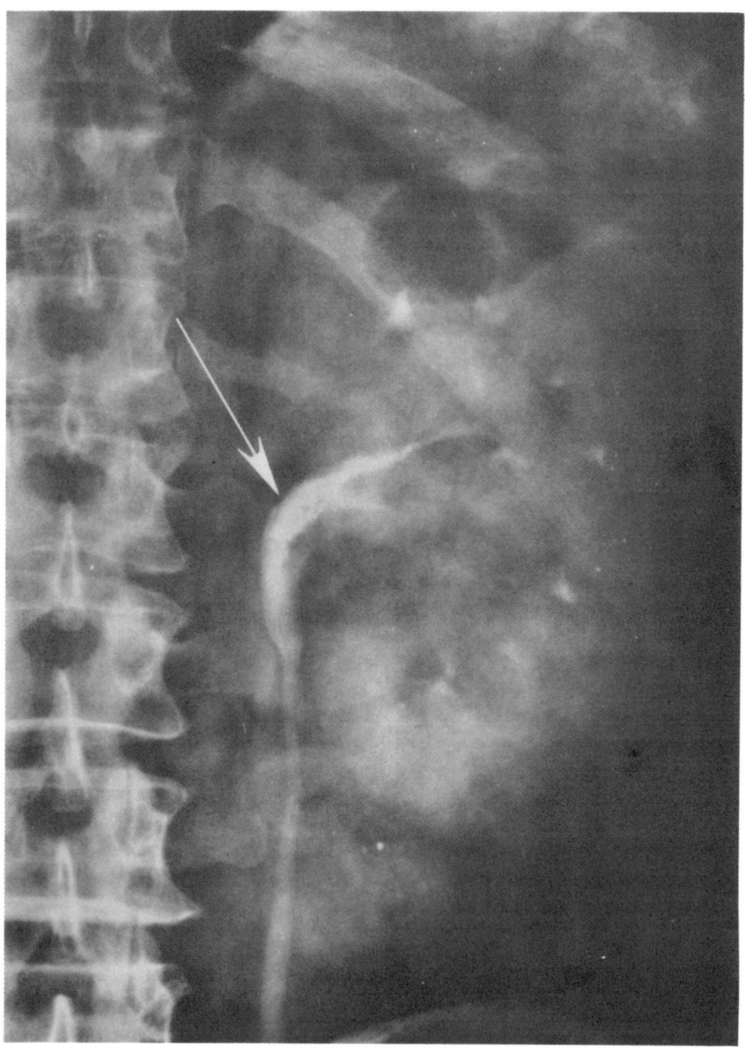

Fig. 5 Excretory urogram in renal vein thrombosis. Note enlarged kidney, attenuation of infundibula, and scalloped ureter (arrow) from extrinsic compression by enlarged venous collateral vessels.

The most common complications are self-limited gross hematuria and clinically recognizable perirenal hematoma. Both of these most often can be managed conservatively with bed rest and maintenance of a generous urine volume. Complications are more frequent in patients with moderately advanced renal insufficiency or long-standing hypertension. The mortality rate directly related to a percutaneous renal biopsy procedure is now less than 0.2%, again in experienced hands. When there is a contraindication to the use of percutaneous renal biopsy (for example, in the presence of a solitary or horseshoe kidney or gross coagulation abnormalities), open renal biopsy is the procedure of choice. The surgical team, however, must have available the appropriate fixative solutions, some of which are not routinely used in the preparation of surgical specimens. Usually, a wedge section is obtained in lieu of a biopsy needle core.

Whether one uses measurements from a kidney-ureter-bladder roentgenogram or an excretory urogram or utilizes the fluoroscopic technique for kidney localization seems to make little difference in the success rate of obtaining adequate tissue by the percutaneous technique. Inexperienced operators or those who have been trained in recent years tend to prefer fluoroscopic aid in kidney localization; this adds to the expense of the procedure and sometimes may not be technically applicable in patients with poor renal function. In biopsy situations that predictably are technically difficult, such as pronounced obesity or severe spinal deformity, fluoroscopy should be considered the technique of choice, however. Patients with the recent onset of moderately severe and uncontrolled hypertension in whom renal biopsy is considered urgent are best managed by parenterally administered antihypertensive medications (for example, diazoxide or nitroprusside) given shortly before and after the procedure. The recently available potent oral agent minoxidil should diminish the occasions when the former two antihypertensive drugs are necessary.

Patients who consent to the procedure of percutaneous renal biopsy should be appraised of the potential risks, complications, chance of unsuccessful outcome, and the realization that a diagnosis may not result in any specific therapy that is known to be effective. Physicians who regularly do renal biopsy generally find it less difficult to maintain expertise in their technique and are more successful in consistently providing adequate tissue for examination. Inadequate tissue is tantamount to no tissue.

Preparation of the renal tissue is extremely important. Unless a well-defined lesion is seen in a single available glomerulus or vessel, a minimum of five glomeruli is usually considered necessary for adequate biopsy specimen interpretation. Even then, some focal diseases can be missed through sampling error. Preparation of tissue and morphologic interpretation are best performed by a pathologist who maintains an interest in renal diseases and who has continuing access to a generous volume of renal biopsy material.

For achieving optimal information, the pathologist must use all three of the currently available techniques for tissue examination: light microscopy, immunofluorescence, and electron microscopy. Each may add significant information in the overall diagnostic assessment. Thin-section (2- to 3-μm) light microscopy utilizing hematoxylin and eosin, periodic acid-Schiff, silver methenamine, and other tissue stains requires continual quality control by experienced laboratory technicians. Indirect immunofluorescent staining techniques now routinely use fluorescein-tagged antibodies to immunoglobulins IgG, IgA, and IgM, complement, fibrinogen, and sometimes properdin. Electron microscopy is the third technique considered essential for the optimal evaluation of renal tissue. As with light microscopy and immunofluorescent staining, electron microscopy adds to the total pathologic appraisal and, like the others, is especially helpful in some diseases—for example, the early stages of membranous glomerulopathy in which lesions may be scattered but very specific when seen.

Obviously, adequate tissue is a more difficult objective to achieve when all three techniques are used; very careful attention must be directed to the allotment of glomeruli-containing tissue for each fixative. Newer methods, now in development, should allow light microscopy, immunofluorescent staining, and electron microscopy examination to be performed on a singly fixed specimen.

Despite adequate tissue preparation and interpretation, the pathologist often finds it difficult to make a specific clinical diagnosis after renal tissue examination. His interpretation does provide information helpful in establishing a limited differential diagnosis of disease processes known to be associated with the morphologic description. In the same way, the clinician will have information that alerts the pathologist to possible diagnoses so that special techniques of tissue examination and careful search for focal morphologic abnormalities are pursued.

The pathologist, with information from the clinician, may find it necessary to use additional staining techniques to clarify the tissue diagnosis. This is particularly true when amyloidosis is suspected, because the staining properties of amyloid deposition vary considerably. Congo red, methyl violet, and thioflavin-T preparations are valuable when amyloidosis is a consideration. Electron microscopy is the most definitive technique, with amyloid fibrils being unique in appearance.

For physicians who perform renal biopsies and who do not have readily available pathology support for tissue processing and interpretation, it is now possible to conveniently send biopsy specimens to laboratories where this can be done with good quality control. Ideally, however, the patient is best served when clinician and pathologist are closely associated.

Special Studies

Special laboratory studies are often dictated by the renal changes noted on examination of biopsy tissue, as well as by the clinical characteristics presented by the patient. Again, good communication is needed between the clinician and pathologist in order to properly evaluate the nephrotic patient.

When amyloidosis is suspected, rectal biopsy tissue is much easier and safer to procure than renal tissue. In experience at our institution with nephrosis secondary to renal amyloidosis, rectal tissue is positive for amyloid in about 60% to 70% of cases.

The serum levels of whole complement, obtained as part of the basic nephrotic workup, can be decreased in several clinical settings:[23] (1) acute poststreptococcal glomerulonephritis; (2) idiopathic membranoproliferative glomerulonephritis (70%); (3) active systemic lupus erythematosus; (4) subacute bacterial endocarditis; (5) infected ventriculoatrial or peritoneal shunts; (6) nonspecific vasculitis (occasionally); and (7) essential mixed cryoglobulinemia. Thus, additional special studies in the presence of low levels of serum whole complement might include (1) further evaluation for systemic lupus erythematosus with antinative DNA determination, lupus erythematosus clot test, and skin biopsy; (2) special serum protein studies; and (3) blood cultures if an associated fever, disproportionate anemia, or heart murmur is noted.

The determination of serum cryoglobulin level is appropriate in the presence of unusual skin lesions, especially when the pathologist notes biopsy features suggestive of a mixed cryo-globulin glomerular injury. Blood specimens should be collected in a syringe and clotted in tubes, both of which are maintained at body temperature. When coagulation is allowed to occur at room temperature, some cryoglobulin may be precipitated with the clot.

Hepatitis B_S antigen has been found with membranous glomerulopathy as well as with the vasculitides.[24,25] The clinical significance of this antigen presence is as yet not clear, and there is no currently recognized relationship between hepatitis and any type or stage of the various glomerulopathies.

One of the pulmonary-renal syndromes, Goodpasture's syndrome, and some instances of idiopathic rapidly progressive glomerulonephritis produce a linear fluorescent staining pattern along the capillary basement membrane with fluorescein-tagged anti-IgG.[26] This is strong evidence for a glomerular injury mechanism mediated by antibodies formed against glomerular basement-membrane antigen. When this immunofluorescent pattern is seen, further support of a diagnosis can be gained by the detection of circulating serum antiglomerular basement-membrane antibodies. Techniques for detecting these circulating antibodies to glomerular basement-membrane antigen are available in many renal pathology laboratories. The absence of these antibodies, however, does not completely rule out either of these diagnoses.[27] The usefulness of this test in patient management will be discussed later.

Angiography may be an additional special radiographic procedure used in the patient with suspected renal vein thrombosis. (Clinical clues that suggest this diagnosis have been previously mentioned.) This complication seems to occur more frequently in nephrotic patients with membranous glomerulopathy.[28] The parenchymal renal disease precedes the vein thrombosis; however, it is unclear as to why these patients with membranous renal lesions appear to be at greater risk than other nephrotic patients. Coagulation abnormalities generally occur in most nephrotic patients,[1] but as yet, no different clotting abnormalities have been noted in those patients with renal vein thrombosis.[29]

Although renal venography can easily detect inferior vena cava occlusion with thrombosis, the detection of thrombosis limited to the renal veins is subject to considerable errors with this technique. In our institution, renal arteriography is first performed to outline any possible renal masses and to visualize the main renal vein during late sequence films. This is followed by an injection of epinephrine into the renal artery and a subsequent retrograde injection of contrast medium into the renal vein via a femoral vein catheter. Although this technique is more complicated, it is much superior in outlining the renal venous system, especially the smaller venous radicles not visualized with venography alone.

Chapter 4

APPROACH TO DIURESIS

The edema formation of nephrosis, in itself, seldom is a life-threatening condition. It does cause considerable morbidity in terms of discomfort, lack of mobility, susceptibility to dermal infections, complications of wound healing, cosmetic appearance, aggravation of incisional hernias, and, in the presence of pleural effusions, significant dyspnea. The primary objective in implementing diuresis in the nephrotic patient is not to eliminate edema formation but to lessen morbidity through attainment of an acceptable degree of extracellular fluid retention. Frequently, patients with newly diagnosed nephrotic syndrome have accumulated fluid so insidiously that they are not fully aware of its extent. Loss of weight from excessive breakdown of muscle protein is replaced by gain in weight from the formation of edema. For this reason, the patient's actual gain in weight considerably misrepresents the amount of fluid accumulation.

Not all nephrotic patients are edematous to a degree that requires correction. The physician must determine this in each situation. A point to remember is the increased tissue laxity present in older adults compared with young patients and, therefore, the tendency for older adults to manifest edema more readily in the presence of similar degrees of hypoalbuminemia. Some patients may retain edema fluid comprising 15 to 20% of their total body weight when in the nephrotic state.

Certain obvious states of edema require more prompt alleviation than others. Ascites (by limitation of diaphragmatic excursion), pleural effusion (by decreased lung expansion to the point of dyspnea), and pedal edema (enough to cause fluid loss through skin breakdown) are a few of the more common situations of immediate concern. In obese patients particularly, edema formation may add to the technical problems of performing a percutaneous renal biopsy. When an open renal biopsy is

considered to be the procedure of choice, the incision necessary for kidney exposure is subject to poor healing and subsequent infection if edema is severe.

Although only a temporary measure, thoracentesis may be
necessary for relief of dyspnea when a large pleural effusion is
present. Fortunately, the occurrence of pulmonary edema in
the nephrotic patient is uncommon. When it occurs, it is
usually the result of (1) hypertensive cardiac disease; (2) amyloid cardiac infiltration; or (3) unsuccessful diuretic efforts
with mannitol or serum albumin. In the patient with refractory
oliguria whose renal function is insufficient to effectively re-
move these agents, the abrupt increase in plasma oncotic pressure may precipitate acute pulmonary edema. In the latter cir-
cumstance, a greater-than-normal vascular volume rapidly develops with the concurrent improvement of vascular oncotic
pressure as extracellular, extravascular fluid is redistributed
into the vascular space at a rate faster than that which can be
effectively removed by renal excretion. Thus, if no diuresis
occurs, this iatrogenic complication may be sustained and ne-
cessitate emergency phlebotomy or dialysis (or both).

The initial diuresis of the nephrotic patient is best managed
in a hospital setting, where close monitoring of fluid intake and
urine output, body weight, and vital signs can be achieved.
Among the factors to consider at the onset of diuretic attempts
are (1) level of renal function; (2) degree of hypoalbuminemia;
(3) blood pressure; (4) past symptoms suggestive of cardiovascular disorders, such as unstable angina and transient cerebral ischemic attacks; and (5) orthostatic hypotensive tendencies from peripheral neuropathy (as experienced by some patients with diabetes or amyloidosis).

These considerations are of importance, primarily because
of the potential dangers they present when the diuresis course
is not optimal; they will be discussed subsequently in relation
to the means of promoting fluid removal.

Activity

Although many nephrotic patients show modest spontaneous diuretic tendencies when kept at bed rest, moderate ambulation
should be encouraged. As mentioned previously, the abnormal
clotting factors present in nephrotic patients are a potential
cause of thromboembolic events that may be enhanced by immobilization. Increased susceptibility to infections, combined

with poor ventilatory mechanics and a tendency toward aspiration pneumonia when eating at bed rest, also argues against enforced immobilization.

Accurate Observation of Vital Signs and Weight

A record of daily weight is perhaps the best guideline for the appropriate rate of diuresis. Uncomfortably edematous patients can safely lose 2 to 5 lb (1.4 to 2.3 kg) per day initially. This rate should decrease as the desired weight is approached, however. The rate of diuresis and a suitable end point also depend on adjustments of vascular volume, which is best monitored by determinations of supine and upright blood pressures taken several times daily.

Older patients who undergo diuresis too rapidly may suffer serious hypotension, with resultant myocardial or cerebral damage. Likewise, any nephrotic patient with an associated disease that may cause sympathetic nervous dysfunction will require close observation and the taking of standing blood pressure because of an exaggerated tendency toward orthostatic hypotension. Patients with diabetes mellitus or amyloidosis represent the most common examples of this.

Excessively rapid diuresis can precipitate acute renal failure. In the presence of a brisk diuresis, even close observation of changes in edema may be misleading to the physician, because of the delay in fluid equilibration between vascular and extravascular compartments. A modestly sustained or sometimes interrupted diuresis ideally allows the managing physician to obtain a more reliable estimate of the patient's dry weight. This is frequently considerably less than the "usual" weight that is familiar to the patient.

Diet, Fluid Intake, and Output

Effective communication between the physician and a dietician who is well acquainted with low-sodium diets is essential for an efficient, successful diuretic program in the initial management of a nephrotic patient. Edematous nephrotic patients frequently have a sensation of abdominal fullness and experience discomfort secondary to ascites and gastrointestinal edema which decreases their desire for many types of foods. Periodic reassessment by the dietician of the hospitalized patient's eating habits helps to assure optimal nutrition under what sometimes are prolonged and difficult circumstances.

Dietary modifications used during an aggressive diuresis program can be much more strict than those used during a chronic maintenance program. In-hospital diets containing 20 to 25 meq of sodium should be readily available, whereas patients are seldom willing or able to follow such rigid dietary sodium restrictions when eating at home. During difficult conditions of diuresis, that is, in patients with renal insufficiency and low levels of serum albumin, a strict control of dietary sodium may make the difference between a reasonable hospital stay and one that is prolonged because of indolent edema. The protein content in a 25-meq sodium diet is, by necessity, limited to approximately 50 to 60 g, but over a short time, this limitation of protein does not adversely affect the already diminished levels of serum albumin. Most dietetic kitchens can provide a reasonably palatable menu with such sodium restriction. The use of sodium substitutes, usually potassium chloride, is not generally well accepted by patients. These substitutes require that they be added just before the ingestion of each food portion and they also tend to leave an unpleasant metallic aftertaste. Lemon juice seems to be a more suitable flavoring substitute.

Too often, little consideration is given to the total daily fluid intake during diuresis, a factor that, if unheeded, may greatly limit the success of a diuretic program. Generally, patients should be limited to a total 24-hr fluid intake (including water in food) of between 1,200 and 1,500 ml. Even more stringent restrictions may be necessary under difficult conditions. Urine volume should be monitored and charted for each voiding, along with the patient's daily prebreakfast weight. This information will be valuable in determining the effectiveness of the individual doses of diuretic agent.

Diuretic Medications and Oncotic Agents

Before discussing the use of diuretic agents, a review of renal sodium handling and of renal tubule sites of diuretic agent action is in order.

Of the total 24-hr filtered water (144 liters) and sodium (20,000 meq), 70% is reabsorbed in the proximal renal tubule (Fig. 6, site 1). The thick ascending limb of the loop of Henle and the cortical diluting segment (sites 2 and 3) are capable of reabsorbing 50 to 75% of the balance of tubular fluid sodium and chloride. This is accomplished without accompanying fluid reabsorption. The remaining tubular fluid sodium can be reabsorbed at site 4 in the distal convoluted tubule and, unlike in the

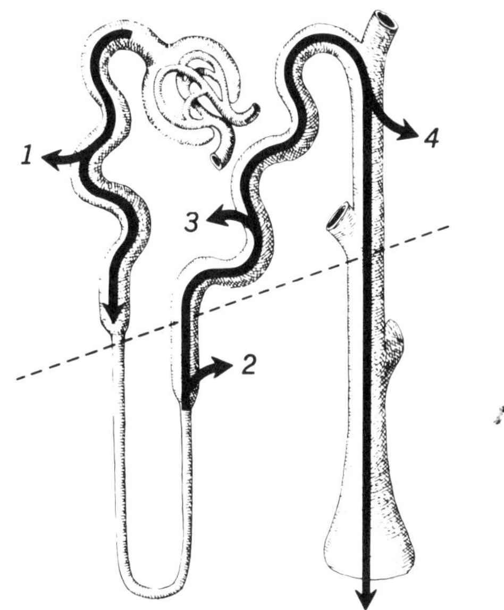

Fig. 6 Sites of renal tubular sodium reabsorption: (1) proximal
      renal tuble; (2) medullary diluting segment; (3) cortical
      diluting segment; (4) distal renal tubule. (From Searle
      Pharmaceuticals, Inc., Aldosterone in Clinical Practice
      [monograph], Chicago, 1974. Reprinted by per-
      mission.)

three other sites, the sodium is exchanged for potassium. Site
4 is under the influence of the hormone aldosterone. There are
two factors that influence sodium reabsorption at this most distal site 4: (1) the amount of sodium delivered to the site and (2)
the amount of aldosterone available. For the first three sites,
only factor (1) is influential. In the presence of the nephrotic
syndrome, aldosterone production is extremely high. In fact,
except for the clinical conditions of primary aldosterone-se-
creting adrenal tumor and adrenal hyperplasia, the nephrotic
syndrome is characteristically associated with some of the high-
est aldosterone production levels found in edematous states.

For each of the four sites of sodium reabsorption, diuretic
medications are available in the clinician's armamentarium
(Fig. 6). Site 1, the proximal renal tubule where the greatest
reabsorption occurs, is influenced by acetazolamide. Unfortunately, the amount of sodium reabsorption blocked by this

agent is so minimal that the drug has almost no use in an effective diuretic program.

Site 2, the medullary diluting segment (thick ascending limb of the loop of Henle), is influenced by the loop diuretic agents furosemide and ethacrynic acid.[30,31] These agents are extremely effective sodium-reabsorptive blocking agents and are the mainstay of the initial diuretic program in most nephrotic patients. Their effectiveness is limited primarily by the amount of sodium and chloride delivered to the medullary diluting segment of the renal tubule.

Site 3, the cortical diluting segment, is influenced by thiazide diuretics. In mildly edematous states, this class of diuretic agents may be sufficient when used alone, or in the presence of refractory edema, these agents may be additive in action to the loop diuretics furosemide and ethacrynic acid.

Although all thiazides appear to act at the same site in the nephron, their duration of action is variable. While chlorothiazide and hydrochlorothiazide have a duration of action of 6 to 12 hr, the drug metolazone is effective in a single daily dose regimen. With renal function levels less than 30% of normal, the short-acting thiazides appear to be relatively ineffective;[32] however, the longer-acting agents seem to maintain some potency.

For sodium reabsorptive blockage at site 4, the distal renal tubule (cortical collective duct), spironolactone remains the primary agent.[33]

Some nephrotic patients require only a moderate amount of less potent diuretic medication for optimal diuresis. An outpatient program consisting of a combination diuretic and potassium-sparing agent such as Aldactazide (spironolactone and hydrochlorothiazide), two to four tablets daily, will suffice in patients whose edema is mild and whose renal function is normal or minimally reduced. Patients who require a more aggressive approach should be hospitalized, where, in addition to measures discussed previously, therapy should be started with the aldosterone-blocking agent spironolactone in a dose of 25 to 50 mg four times a day.

One of the most common clinical disorders associated with very high levels of aldosterone production is nephrosis. As previously discussed, aldosterone production is a response to hypovolemia induced by decreased plasma oncotic pressure and has no adequate shutoff mechanism—the retained sodium and water continually shifting into the extracellular compartment. Not until serum albumin levels are restored to normal will the stimulus cease for the excessive production of aldosterone. Spironolactone alone is seldom sufficient to promote a satisfactory diuresis because it can only block the absorption of sodium delivered to the distal renal tubules (discussed previously). A diminished load of filtered sodium at the glomerular level and the subsequent increased proximal tubular reabsorption provide little sodium available for blockage at this distal site. In fact, in some untreated nephrotic patients, the kidney has such an avidity for sodium reabsorption that 24-hr urine levels of 20 meq or less are common.

Spironolactone also provides a secondary function that is necessary during aggressive diuresis, that is, potassium sparing. Loop diuretics, such as furosemide and ethacrynic acid, and the thiazides produce excessive loss of body potassium stores by effectively delivering more sodium to distal tubular exchange sites, where tubular fluid sodium is exchanged for potassium. Spironolactone, by blocking the aldosterone-influenced sodium reabsorption at this site, diminishes the effective exchange of potassium for sodium.

Spironolactone should be cautiously used in patients with modest renal insufficiency, and either the drug should not be used or the dosage decreased in patients with serum creatinine levels of 3 mg/dl or greater because of the potential development of serious hyperkalemia. The maximal effect of spironolactone is not reached for 1 to 2 days, so the vigorous use of other diuretics that have a kaliuretic effect might best be delayed for 24 hr. Side effects of the drug are uncommon. Nausea may occur; and gynecomastia may develop, but this does not present a problem with short-term use.

A loop diuretic such as furosemide or ethacrynic acid is next added. Oral furosemide therapy is started, beginning with a single dose of 40 mg. If the urine volume does not increase within 2 hr, the dose should be increased to 80 or 120 mg and the effect observed. Unless the effects of individual doses are periodically monitored, one may continue with inadequate amounts of the diuretic and waste costly hospital time for the patient. Once an effective dose is reached, it can be repeated two or three times daily, but the parameters discussed previously should always be closely monitored. A common error for the physician who manages the diuresis is to prescribe a diuretic dosage schedule for 1 or 2 days without observing short-term results of the program.

Occasionally, patients may require, two or three times daily, oral doses of furosemide which are greater than 120 mg. Often these are patients whose renal function is greatly depressed. Orally administered furosemide may not be well tolerated, especially producing upper gastrointestinal symptoms at higher dosage levels. Decreased absorption, possibly from gastrointestinal edema, is a second problem. If these situations are suspected, the intravenous administration of the drug is substituted, but the initial dosage should be small and the influence on urine volume observed before considering a larger dose. Intravenously administered furosemide is given as a bolus during a 5-min period, and the increase in urine volume should be apparent within 30 to 60 sec. Hearing loss has been observed in some patients given large intravenous doses of furosemide,[34] and the impairment may be irreversible. Sometimes after the initial bolus, a continuous infusion of furosemide (80 to 400 mg in 500 ml of 5% dextrose and water given at 100 ml/hr) will result in a sustained diuresis.

To facilitate the effect of the aldosterone-blocking agent and of the loop diuretic, serum albumin may be added to the diuretic program. The immediate effect of an osmotic agent is an increase in vascular volume, improvement of renal plasma flow and glomerular filtration rate, and an increase in the delivery of filtered sodium to tubular sites where diuretic agents exert their action. With difficult diuresis, 100 ml of a 25% solution of salt-free serum albumin are given intravenously during a 30- to 60-min period. This is followed by the intravenous administration of furosemide. Much of the administered albumin is shortly lost by urinary excretion, but its temporary improvement of effective intravascular oncotic pressure is not uncommonly followed by a sustained improvement in diuresis. Additional use of serum albumin is then usually unnecessary. Daily decisions about further serum albumin administration is an individual matter, however.

For the nephrotic patient who is being prepared for surgery, serum albumin is used more aggressively, both to improve plasma oncotic pressure and to promote wound healing. The presence of renal insufficiency should not be a deterrent to utilizing serum albumin intravenously for fear of precipitating gross clinical uremia because the added protein effect is only transient. The greatest danger with the use of serum albumin is the precipitation of acute pulmonary edema. In elderly patients, patients with borderline cardiac status, and patients who are not likely to have a prompt diuresis, caution is necessary when using this means to facilitate increased urine output.

Mannitol is seldom used as an osmotic diuretic in nephrotic patients anymore because of the potent diuretic drug armamentarium now available to the clinician.

Electrolyte and Renal Function Monitoring

Clinically significant electrolyte abnormalities will not occur if the person managing the nephrotic diuresis has prescience of potential problems. Alterations in serum sodium and chloride levels occur infrequently when the previously discussed diuretic program is used. Excessive water intake on rare occasions is enough to produce symptomatic hyponatremia (serum Na < 120 meq/dl) and is best managed by the rigid restriction of oral and intravenous fluid.

Despite the use of spironolactone and loop diuretic agents, clinically significant urinary potassium losses may occur. Because the diuresis in this instance is brief, potassium losses are usually reflected by serum potassium levels. Prolonged diuresis at a slower rate, however, permits a more gradual intercompartmental shift of potassium, which is not always reflected in serum potassium levels. A serum potassium determination every 2 to 3 days during diuresis should detect any unexpected major problems of hypokalemia. If concern exists about the effect of hypokalemia, electrocardiographic monitoring should forewarn of the most serious complication, which is cardiac arrhythmia. Potassium supplements are seldom necessary during diuresis when spironolactone is used, but for nephrotic patients who are taking digitalis, close monitoring of serum potassium levels and electrocardiographic tracings is important to detect the need for potassium supplements.

Metabolic alkalosis during forced diuresis also may become a problem. Because relatively more choloride than sodium is excreted during diuresis, increased amounts of potassium and hydrogen ions, the latter in the form of NH_4 and titratable acids, are required to accompany the chloride anion. Also contributing to the alkalosis is a relative extracellular volume depletion which is sensed by the kidney, initiating increased proximal tubular reabsorption of filtered bicarbonate.[35] In the presence of alkalosis, hypokalemia is accentuated as potassium in extracellular fluid shifts intracellularly to replace the depleted hydrogen ion storage. Potassium chloride is used in the treatment of this combined hypokalemia and hypochloremic metabolic alkalosis. If fluids are to be employed, the intravenous route may be used. If not, oral potassium chloride syrup (20 meq potassium per 15 ml) is used three times daily, with careful serial potassium monitoring.

Serum uric acid levels become a problem for patients with renal insufficiency or a history of gout who are given potent loop diuretics. Although most patients with renal insufficiency do not develop acute gouty arthritis when moderate elevations of serum uric acid level occur, some attain serum levels greater than 11 mg/dl. There are some clinicians who recommend the use of a xanthine oxidase inhibitor when levels greater than 11 mg/dl develop during diuresis. In the patient with a known history of gout, allopurinol should be given before diuresis is begun if the drug is not already a part of the patient's program. The dosage should be decreased in the presence of renal insufficiency to minimize possible side effects.

Laboratory assessment of renal function, as judged by the level of serum creatinine, should be done every 2 or 3 days during vigorous diuresis. Patients with renal insufficiency are likely to have transient elevations in serum creatinine levels, and a rare patient may develop signs of uremia. Loop and thiazide diuretics have been reported to cause an acute interstitial nephritis,[36-38] a factor to be considered if a large increase in serum creatinine level occurs during diuresis. These diuretics should be discontinued when a hypersensitivity reaction is suspected and daily serum creatinine determinations then obtained. In most cases of this complication, there are no other clues, such as fever or eosinophilia, which are helpful, and because the patient usually has just undergone renal biopsy, it is difficult to justify doing a subsequent procedure, so close temporally, to support the diagnosis. Recently, gallium scanning of the kidneys has been reported to be of aid in diagnosing interstitial nephritis.[39]

An adverse effect from contrast medium also may strikingly increase serum creatinine levels. This complication fortunately is transient, oliguria subsiding within 3 to 7 days and the serum creatinine decreasing to preexposure levels in about the same time duration.

Other possible reasons for the increasing serum creatinine levels during diuresis are the precipitation of renal vein thrombosis from vascular volume depletion or acute renal failure secondary to a rapid and sustained reduction in renal perfusion.

Perhaps of more value than any previously discussed single guideline during diuresis of the nephrotic patient is the daily review by the clinician of his projected goal. The end result should be a diuresis accompanied by a few symptoms and uncomplicated by any of the potential problems discussed.

Chapter 5

LONG-TERM MANAGEMENT

Dietary and Diuretic Approaches

Most adult patients with the nephrotic syndrome unfortunately
have types of renal disease for which there is no successful
specific therapy, and as a result they must adjust to problems
attendant upon chronic heavy proteinuria as well as those common to any type of chronic renal disease without nephrosis.
Foremost among these problems is the management of edema,
hypertension, chronic renal insufficiency, and hyperlipidemia.

Dietary modifications are the basis of this chronic management approach.[40-42] Once excessive edema has been relieved,
a combination diet and medication program that will best sus-
tain the postdiuresis status can then be established. Again,
close cooperation between the dietician and the clinician is essential. The program best suited for each patient is most
easily accomplished in the hospital after the initial diuresis.
In fact, if the patient's maintenance program is not arranged
and observed in the hospital, future problems of medical control are common. The basic diet for most nephrotic patients
with grossly normal renal function should consist of 60 to 90
meq of sodium and no water restriction. Protein intake, predominantly of high biological value, is kept at a maximum but
within the sodium modification limit.

Dietary management of the nephrotic syndrome is directed
toward control of edema and hypoproteinemia. A high dietary
protein intake (to replace the urinary protein loss), controlled
sodium (to minimize the edema), and adequate calories (to prevent muscle catabolism and to supply an adequate energy
source) are the primary therapeutic goals. The patient's nutritional state and the underlying renal condition must be considered when prescribing the diet. Because many edematous nephrotic patients are also anorexic, particular attention and
supervision should be given to their actual dietary intake.

If renal function is grossly normal, 100 g or more of protein ($1\frac{1}{2}$ to 2 g/kg for adults) per day and adequate calories are indicated (Table 2). Adult men may eat 100 to 140 g of protein per day, and this can be continued over a long period; but women will seldom eat more than 100 g/day. Commercial protein supplements are available for patients who have difficulty consuming these recommended amounts of protein. Dried milk also can be mixed with regular milk to make double-rich milk or with other foods to increase the dietary protein. The dietary protein recommended for nephrotic children is approximately 2 to 3 g/kg of body weight (normal requirement 1.2 to 1.5 g/kg) to allow for both positive nitrogen balance and growth. If renal function is less than 50% of normal, the dietary protein should be modified as for other patients with chronic renal failure, but protein equal to the urinary protein loss is added. Proteins of high biological value (eggs, milk, meat) should be used to supply approximately 75% of the total protein in the diet (Table 2).

Patients who are not obese should receive between 1,800 and 3,500 kcal/day, depending on their height, weight, age, sex, and activity. Weight reduction for the obese patient should be considered but should not be aggressively pursued. A sudden decrease in the amount of calories will only encourage catabolism of body tissue. Because of the need to incorporate generous amounts of protein, weight reduction is best achieved with approximately 1,600 to 1,800 cal. At this level, the diet requires no commercial products and is far more practicable for the patient.

The patient should be encouraged to weigh himself daily and to report to his physician any sudden gain or loss in weight in excess of 5 lb (2.3 kg) since this would indicate a significant change in extracellular fluid. Gain or loss of 1 lb (0.45 kg) of fat requires the addition or reduction of 3,000 to 3,500 cal. Therefore, body tissue weight loss or weight gain should and will be achieved at a slow but steady rate.

After diuresis, control of edema and of the commonly seen complication, hypertension, usually can be achieved by a sodium allowance of 90 meq (2 g) or less per day. Adequate control of dietary sodium decreases diuretic needs and allows the patient to have fluids ad libitum. Care should be taken when requesting the diet so as to avoid confusion between a 90-meq (2-g) sodium diet and a 2-g salt diet, because sodium and salt are not synonymous to the dietician who is planning the diet. In fact, with a 2-g salt diet, the patient would receive approximately

Table 2 Sample Menu for Patients with the Nephrotic Syndrome

Diet of 100 g of protein, 90 meq of sodium, and approximately 2,200 calories

Breakfast

Grapefruit sections　　　　　2 slices whole wheat
1 Fried egg[a]　　　　　　　　　toast
Butter[a]　　　　　　　　　　　Marmalade[b]
1 Cup milk[a]
Coffee or tea, if desired
Mid-morning snack, if desired: Banana

Lunch

Hot sliced turkey (3 oz.) (SF[c]) sandwich
Broccoli spears (SF[c])
Fresh fruit salad with mayonnaise
Slice of old-fashioned pound cake dusted with powdered
　　　sugar[b]
1 Cup milk[a]
Coffee or tea, if desired
Mid-afternoon snack, if desired: Grapes

Dinner

Roast loin of pork[a] (4 oz.) (SF[c]) with spiced apple ring[b]
Boiled potato (SF[c])
Radishes—turnip greens (SF[c])
Corn muffin　　　　　　　　　　Butter[a]
Baked pears with lemon sauce[b]
1 Cup milk[a]
Coffee or tea, if desired
Bedtime snack: Strawberry ice cream with [c]vanilla wafer[a,b]

---

[a]Dietary cholesterol may be decreased by using egg substitute (allow for sodium content), skim milk, margarine, and low-fat desserts.

[b]If free sugars are to be limited, fresh fruits and artificially sweetened desserts should be used. Complex carbohydrates and fats should be increased to compensate for the decrease in calories.

[c]SF denotes prepared without salt. All other spices may be used as desired.

35 meq (1 g) of sodium.   Clarification of salt versus sodium also should be conveyed to the patient.

The control of dietary sodium often has been considered an impossibility when all foods must be prepared at home without the use of commercial products that are low in salt. This, in reality, is not true. Even with the need for increased calories, one usually can include ordinary commercial bread and butter or margarine in the diet. Discussing food preparation techniques used by restaurants aids in teaching patients how to eat out and yet maintain control of their diet.

Most foods contain either natural or added sodium. Once a level of needed sodium is established, the diet should be planned with consideration given to the patient's likes, dislikes, and needs. Most often patients have been consuming "salty" foods which they especially like. The patient should be taught how to compensate for this extra salt eating by selecting for the rest of the day foods that contain very little sodium.

Hypercholesterolemia and hypertriglyceridemia are frequently seen in patients with nephrotic syndrome. The influence that these lipid alterations have on the potential development of atherosclerosis in the nephrotic patient is uncertain. Since these lipid abnormalities are secondary effects, drug therapy (such as use of clofibrate) or stringent dietary restrictions are ineffective in influencing a significant change. There is also the possible danger of precipitating muscle damage with the use of clofibrate in these patients, particularly those with renal insufficiency.

Optimal care requires that patients consume the diets prescribed for them. All too often diets that are high in protein, low in sodium, and high in calories are advised but not consumed. The dietician is invaluable in teaching the patient the importance of the diet by adjusting the diet to the patient's eating habits and, if the patient is hospitalized, in serving the correct diet. With the right planning, diets in which sodium is maintained at a level of 60 to 90 meq can be very palatable. The better the attitude of the staff and the better the teaching, the more effective the patient compliance will be. Explanation of kidney function and its relationship to diet is essential for the patient's understanding. Teaching need not and should not be of a textbook nature. Honesty and simplicity in communicating knowledge of the disease are often the best approach. The patient who understands why he is following a particular diet is most always more cooperative. Emphasizing diet "control" rather than diet "restriction" is an important aspect in creating a positive attitude toward diet.

Communication of dietary knowledge should begin early during the course of the patient's stay, whether in a hospital or an outpatient setting. The hospital meals provide an excellent opportunity for the day-to-day teaching of the nutritional part of the management program. With good diet planning and teaching, the patient can return home with a positive, workable attitude of dietary control.

Provided the patient adheres to his recommended diet, the average nephrotic patient needs to take only a combination of a thiazide and a potassium-sparing diuretic two to three times daily for effective control of edema. On occasion, when there is a lapse in the dietary salt restriction and a gain in weight, diuretic supplementation with furosemide for 2 to 3 consecutive days or three times weekly will suffice for readjustment. Patients will often learn how to manipulate these supplemental diuretics themselves, recognizing that a certain drug dosage will produce a predictable reduction in weight.

Nephrotic patients with very low serum albumin levels usually have edema that is not easily controlled; these patients should use spironolactone daily plus furosemide once or twice daily. They may also need to supplement their diuretic program at times with increased amounts of furosemide. A greater degree of chronic edema must be accepted unless in occasional patients the serum albumin level can be increased by a sustained effort to maintain the dietary protein intake over 90 g/day. This amount of dietary protein is frequently difficult to achieve by the patient, however.

As renal function declines, and it will in most adult nephrotic patients, higher doses of a thiazide or a change to furosemide will be required to control the edema. A reassessment of dietary sodium intake is helpful also, the sodium content being decreased to between 40 and 60 meq/day. With some renal diseases, heavy proteinuria diminishes, along with renal function deterioration, and therefore, the edema becomes easier to control with the same amount of salt restriction. Continuing heavy proteinuria and decreasing renal function create a major management problem. Because of the need of a protein-restricted diet to prevent clinical uremia and because of their continuing heavy proteinuria, these patients are in such a negative protein balance that adequate nutrition is impossible. Occasionally, in this situation a patient will require bilateral nephrectomy and be entered into a chronic hemodialysis or transplant program at a stage earlier than usual in the course of renal function deterioration. In a few patients who are too ill to undergo nephrectomy, medical nephrectomy by means of an absorbable gelatin sponge (Gelfoam) injected into the renal artery or mercury injected into the renal arteries has been used also, but with limited success.[43,44]

Hypertension Management

Hypertension is not common early during the course of a nephrotic patient's renal disease but very often develops later. The well-accepted fact of accelerated vascular disease and the increased incidence of vascular accidents in the presence of poorly controlled hypertension are now compelling reasons for aggressive efforts to control this complication. Specific treatment programs for the renal diseases that cause nephrosis sometimes include the use of high-dose steroids, a definite aggravating factor of secondary hypertension. This form of hypertension is especially difficult to control satisfactorily. Fortunately, high-dose steroid programs are of relatively short duration in the treatment of most renal diseases. Hypertension treatment programs currently are rightly more concerned with successful blood pressure control than with the often necessary reduction in renal function that accompanies the use of agents that lower blood pressure. Since most nephrotic patients are potential candidates for chronic hemodialysis programs or renal transplantation, the major emphasis in hypertension therapy is in diminishing the risks of vascular complications and not in maintaining maximal renal function. In other words, hypertension should be optimally controlled and the secondary potential consequences of reduced renal perfusion and progressive renal function deterioration accepted as a necessary compromise.

The dietary and medication measures discussed previously form the basis of hypertension therapy in nephrotic patients who have normal or minimally reduced renal function. Several choices for additional medications are available. The most common include methyldopa, hydralazine, propranolol, and metoprolol. The dosage of these drugs should be adjusted accordingly, as is done with any hypertensive patient who does not have the nephrotic syndrome. When renal function reaches a level of 30% or less, short-acting thiazide drugs become less effective for control of edema and hypertension.[45] Then furosemide, combined with any of the previously mentioned drugs and accompanied by dietary sodium restriction, becomes the mainstay in the control of blood pressure. With refractory hypertension, one may choose to try the newer agent minoxidil,[46] realizing, however, that this vasodilating drug is a potent sodium retainer and often requires large amounts of furosemide as a diuretic.

Serum Lipid Management

Some data suggest that cardiovascular complications develop at an earlier age in the nephrotic patient, whether or not hypertension accompanies the syndrome.[47] This is difficult to substantiate because the primary renal disease itself usually shortens the life span of the nephrotic patient. The vascular disease risk factor associated with hypercholesterolemia and hypertriglyceridemia is even more difficult to assess. Little attention has been directed toward control of these lipid abnormalities in the nephrotic patient, primarily because dietary measures alone have such little influence in altering elevations of serum cholesterol and triglyceride levels. Some foods that are high in protein value and low in salt content unfortunately contain generous amounts of cholesterol—for example, eggs. These foods are an important part of the nephrotic diet which, if eliminated, restrict the dietician's choices in devising an appropriate menu. Additionally, when renal insufficiency is advanced enough to require the restriction of protein, total calorie intake is maintained by the substitution of sugars, a dietary element known to aggravate hypertriglyceridemia.

The cholesterol-lowering agent clofibrate is used by some clinicians who treat nephrotic patients, but not enough data have accumulated to support its effectiveness in preventing vascular complications. The drug does lower the levels of serum cholesterol somewhat. However, care should be used in prescribing the drug in the presence of hypoalbuminemia, especially when accompanied by renal insufficiency, because of an increased incidence of side effects.[48] Obviously, further data must be accumulated before one can determine the necessity for controlling hyperlipidemia that accompanies the nephrotic syndrome.

Chapter 6

SPECIFIC TREATMENT OF RENAL DISEASE

Successful treatment of renal diseases responsible for the nephrotic syndrome unfortunately is the exception rather than the
rule. Multiple types of renal lesions and many etiologic factors produce a common syndrome with few clinical features
distinct enough to identify a specific cause without the aid of
special laboratory studies. The clinician and pathologist,
therefore, must by historical information, clinical data, and
study of renal structure either identify a cause or characterize morphologically the renal disease before a specific treatment program can be considered.

When factors such as infections (for example, bacterial endocarditis) or exogenous toxins (for example, mercury, gold,[49]
or D-penicillamine) are identified, appropriate therapy for the
infection or elimination of the toxin constitutes the primary
treatment approach. In most instances, this effort results in
remission of the nephrotic syndrome (although the renal lesion
may persist).[50] For the systemic diseases, therapy directed
at control of that specific disease is also the treatment appropriate for the associated renal lesion. This will be discussed
in more detail later. For the treatment of primary renal diseases, structural classification of the renal lesion itself is of
paramount importance because of the paucity of laboratory data
helpful in distinguishing one "renal disease" from another.

Before individual treatment programs are discussed, men-
tion should be made of a frequently found structural renal lesion—membranous glomerulopathy—which is commonly associated with the nephrotic syndrome but is found in numerous
clinical conditions (Table 3). Familiarity with the differential
diagnosis of this lesion may simplify the clinician's approach
to evaluation and treatment of some nephrotic patients. Because
the disorders listed in Table 3 which can occur with this lesion
also may produce renal lesions other than the membranous
type, the table has its limitations as an all-inclusive differential diagnostic aid.

Table 3 Clinical Disorders Associated with Membranous
Glomerulopathy

---

1. Idiopathic
2. Systemic lupus erythematosus
3. Solid tumor
4. Hepatitis B antigenemia
5. Diabetes mellitus
6. Mercury, gold, and penicillamine
7. Syphilis, malaria
8. Renal vein thrombosis

From large medical centers using current diagnostic criteria, enough data have accumulated to provide a general sta-
tistical breakdown of "primary glomerulopathies" responsible
for the nephrotic syndrome. In an adult nephrotic population,
if one excludes systemic diseases such as diabetes mellitus,
amyloidosis, systemic lupus erythematosus, and so forth, the
most common renal lesion is idiopathic membranous glomerulopathy, accounting for approximately 40% of total cases; lipoid
nephrosis or "nil lesion" disease accounts for 15%, focal
sclerosing glomerulopathy for 15%, membranoproliferative
glomerulonephritis for 15%, and other glomerulonephritides
for 15%.

Idiopathic Membranous Glomerulopathy

Idiopathic membranous glomerulopathy is easily identified
structurally by the pathologist.[51] In its very early stage, however, the lesion may be so focal and subtle that the diagnosis
can be missed unless adequate renal biopsy tissue is available
and carefully examined. It is not known how long this lesion
can be present before producing the nephrotic syndrome—some
patients with milder proteinuria extending over many years
have this lesion. These patients, with asymptomatic proteinuria, may account for 10 to 20% of the total population with
idiopathic membranous glomerulopathy. The natural course of
this disease, when associated with nephrosis, is variable. Several studies have indicated that, with or without treatment attempts using steroids or immunosuppressive drugs (or both),
50 to 75% of patients will reach end-stage renal disease in 10
years.[52,53] Early during the course, hypertension is infrequent. Periodic remissions of the heavy proteinuria are not
uncommon; in fact, about 15 to 20% of adults with idiopathic

membranous glomerulopathy experience a spontaneous remission of the nephrotic syndrome at some time, even though the structural renal lesion invariably persists.[54] Because of this observation, results of treatment programs using prednisone or immunosuppressive agents such as cyclophosphamide (or both) are difficult to interpret.

In 1977, one study reported a favorable influence of high-dose steroid therapy given on an alternate-day schedule for several months, followed by a continuous smaller-dose program indefinitely.[55] The reduction in proteinuria and stabilization of renal function occurred in a much higher percentage of patients than that observed in other studies utilizing shorter courses of steroids. A longer follow-up period will be needed to determine if these observations persist unchanged and if side effects from the long-term use of steroids are acceptable. More recently, preliminary information in a large cooperative study suggests that high-dose steroid therapy for 2 to 3 months, particularly in the presence of an early renal morphologic lesion, may influence proteinuria significantly but, more importantly, may favorably alter the course of progressive renal function deterioration.[56]

At the present time, enough inconsistency exists in our knowledge of the effects of steroids on the course of idiopathic membranous glomerulopathy to withhold judgment about its efficacy until further well-structured treatment programs have been evaluated. As with any proposed treatment program, the risks associated with the use of a medication must be weighed against the possible benefits. Older patients, and those with associated medical conditions such as peptic ulcer, emotional disorders, or osteoporosis, are probably best managed conservatively without a trial of steroids. The most suitable candidate for significant improvement would seem to be the young adult who has a mild renal morphologic lesion. Immunosuppressive drugs alone or in combination with steroids should be avoided because of clearly disappointing past experiences with the former.[57]

As the natural course of disease evolves, heavy proteinuria often diminishes and hypertension and declining renal function become the major management concerns.

Nephrotic syndromes that are associated with solid tumors most commonly have a membranous renal structural lesion. Therefore, patients with idiopathic membranous glomerulopathy should be periodically reassessed for any symptoms suggestive of a malignancy. In one retrospective study, 11% of nephrotic patients developed a malignancy at some time during the course of their renal disease, an incidence considerably higher than what would be expected in the general population.[58] (Experience at our institution suggests that these nephrotic patients have a much lower incidence of malignancy.) Whether or not solid tumors are causative of the nephrotic syndrome is conjectural. Isolated case reports have described tumor-specific antibodies localized in the glomeruli of patients with nephrosis and malignancy;[59] however, further studies of this type of patient are needed before a definite cause-and-effect relationship can be implicated.

Of increasing interest has been the relationship between membranous glomerulopathy and thrombosis of the renal veins. (Abnormalities of clotting factors in nephrotic patients with multiple types of renal lesions have been known for many years, and these seem to be reversible with remission of the syndrome.[60]) The parenchymal renal lesion almost always precedes the thrombosis. Why thrombosis occurs with this renal lesion and not as often with other lesions that cause nephrosis is unclear. One prospective study has observed renal vein thrombosis in 30% of adults with "idiopathic" nephrosis who were studied with renal venography.[28] Many of these patients had histories or urographic abnormalities suggestive of a thromboembolic complication. Experience at our institution suggests that this association is frequent enough (40%) to warrant consideration of angiographic studies in patients who have membranous glomerulopathy, irrespective of symptoms or laboratory findings.[61] Unsuspected renal vein thrombosis definitely occurs and, without angiography, probably will be overlooked.

Treatment of renal vein thrombosis in the presence of nephrosis also has not been well studied. Most specialists in nephrology recommend the use of anticoagulation for an indeterminate time. Again, experience at our institution indicates that clot formation disappears with this treatment approach. Whether it recurs when anticoagulation is stopped is unknown. Certainly, the coagulation defect persists as long as there is heavy proteinuria. While prevention of further thromboembolic complications is the primary consideration,[62] the influence of anticoagulation on the course of the nephrotic syndrome and renal function is still unanswered.

<u>Case Illustrating Renal Vein Thrombosis.</u> A 55-year-old man developed fever and cough, and evidence of an infiltrate was noted on a chest roentgenogram, all of

which cleared gradually without treatment. Two and one-half months later, he noted a gradual gain in weight, then progressive pedal edema. He was hospitalized, diuresed, and given a trial of steroids, but no effect on the initially noted heavy proteinuria was observed. One week after steroid therapy was started, he experienced a left-sided pleuritic pain, followed by hemoptysis and a low-grade fever. A chest infiltrate was again visible on the roentgenogram. The dose of the steroid was reduced gradually during a 10-week period. Three days before his referral, tenderness developed in his left calf.

Physical examination revealed a normal blood pressure, moderate pitting edema of both lower extremities, and deep tenderness in the left calf.

Laboratory studies showed proteinuria (grade 4) and 25 red blood cells, many oval fat bodies, and free lipids per high-power field. The hemoglobin level was normal, serum creatinine 1.2 mg/dl, cholesterol 416 mg/dl, triglycerides 406 mg/dl, serum albumin 1.88 g/dl, and 24-hr urine protein 10.5 g. The roentgenogram of the chest showed no abnormality. Coagulation studies demonstrated an increased fibrinogen level and a strongly positive reaction to the protamine gel test. Findings on the excretory urogram (Fig. 5) indicated renal vein thrombosis. A percutaneous renal biopsy revealed membranous glomerulopathy. A renal venogram demonstrated bilateral thrombosis of the main renal veins, with some evidence of remaining flow compatible with recannulization.

Anticoagulant therapy was started, and the patient was observed periodically during the next 3 years. The edema gradually disappeared, and the use of diuretics and the low-salt diet were discontinued. There were no further episodes of thrombophlebitis or symptoms suggestive of pulmonary emboli. Laboratory studies at the last examination included proteinuria (grade 1), serum creatinine 1.2 mg/dl, and normal levels of serum cholesterol and serum proteins. Anticoagulation was discontinued.

Comment. This patient's history was highly suggestive of renal vein thrombosis complicating the nephrotic syndrome. A history compatible with a pulmonary embolus in any nephrotic patient should create a high suspicion of this complication.[63] Positive urographic findings are rarely found in the presence of renal vein thrombosis. Whether anticoagulation therapy influenced

the course of the renal disease is only conjectural. Findings
on repeat renal biopsy specimens in patients with this type of
course have not been reported. Other patients treated in a
similar fashion have reportedly developed end-stage renal disease, without remission of the nephrotic syndrome.[64]

"Nil Lesion" Nephrosis

Nephrosis associated with a minimal change or "nil lesion" is
more commonly observed in children, accounting for more than
75% of pediatric nephrotic patients.[65] Perhaps 15% of all adult
patients with idiopathic nephrotic syndrome have this disorder.[66] Clinically, the syndrome differs somewhat from nephrosis due to other causes. Initially, hypertension is uncommon, and renal function usually is normal. The urine contains
few if any red cells and no hemoglobin or red cell casts.[67]

Before the diagnosis is made, renal tissue from a biopsy
specimen should be examined by all three techniques previously
mentioned: light microscopy, immunofluorescence, and electron microscopy. The histologic diagnosis basically is made by
a process of elimination. Except for minimal hypercellularity
noted in the glomerular mesangium on light microscopy and a
nonspecific fusion of epithelial cell foot processes seen on electron microscopy, no other morphologic abnormalities are produced by this disorder. Other renal lesions masquerading as
"nil lesion" disease, such as early membranous glomerulopathy, focal sclerosing glomerulonephritis, or mesangioproliferative glomerulonephritis, can be missed if only light microscopy is utilized. Many of the patients described in the earlier
literature who were considered to have "nil lesion" disease and
who did not respond to treatment or who developed end-stage
renal disease probably had other forms of renal disease not
recognized by tissue examination because light microscopy then
was the only technique available.

Although perhaps 20% of patients with the "nil lesion" nephrotic syndrome will experience a spontaneous remission, the
predictable, beneficial effects of steroid therapy have made it
difficult to observe the natural history of this disorder. Since
this disease is present in more than 75% of all nephrotic children, a diagnostic trial of steroids is sometimes used initially;
renal tissue is obtained only if remission of the nephrosis fails
to occur. This practice, however, cannot be supported in nephrotic adults who have no overtly recognizable cause for their
proteinuria because their chance of having a "nil lesion" disorder is considerably less.

A standard treatment program for this disease, once a tissue diagnosis is established, consists of prednisone (60 to 80 mg) in a single daily dose and maintained for a minimum of 1 month. Usually, a reduction in proteinuria begins within 2 to 3 weeks, and with this, the edema disappears. Some physicians prefer to change to an alternate-day dosage schedule when the proteinuria ceases. The dosage of the steroid is then reduced gradually, and its use is discontinued during a period of 2 to 3 months. Patients are instructed to check their urine qualitatively for protein by using the dipstick method. This is the simplest method of detecting, early, any tendency toward a relapse as the dosage of steroid is being reduced gradually.

Four types of steroid response may be expected with this disorder: (1) complete remission, with disappearance of proteinuria, which is sustained; (2) repeated relapses, either during steroid withdrawal or shortly thereafter; (3) reduction in proteinuria to less than 2.0 g/24 hr and associated with an increase in serum albumin level and disappearance of edema formation; and (4) complete lack of response.

In adults, the first type of response is most common, with 60 to 70% of patients experiencing a prolonged remission.[68] If a single relapse occurs at a later date, a similar successful response to therapy can be expected. In patients who experience the second type of response, the so-called steroid-dependent condition, one must consider the possibility of an incorrect diagnosis, as well as the "nil lesion" disorder. Two nephrotic relapses during or shortly after steroid withdrawal characterize the steroid-dependent patient. In this situation, the continued use of high-dose steroids, even on an alternate-day basis, is unjustified and actually, because of steroid side effects, is more harmful than the nephrotic syndrome itself. At this point, the use of a second drug should be considered. Well-controlled studies, with a sufficient follow-up period, have established the effectiveness of a combined drug program for this type of nephrotic patient.[69] Once a nephrotic remission (complete disappearance of urine protein) has been accomplished with prednisone, cyclophosphamide (2 to 3 mg/kg per day orally) is given and its use is continued for a minimum of 2 months. During this time, the dosage of prednisone is reduced gradually and then discontinued. Long-term follow-up studies suggest an expected continued remission rate of at least 50% during a 5-year period.[70] Chlorambucil also has been used in this situation (mainly in Europe), and results similar to those with cyclophosphamide have been obtained.[71] There is understandably some concern regarding the use of these immunosuppressive agents in concern regarding the use of these immunosuppressive agents in a disorder that infrequently is fatal. Although with cyclophosphamide leukopenic bone marrow suppression is not necessary to achieve a prolonged nephrotic remission, leukocyte counts should be taken weekly during this therapy. Hemorrhagic cystitis, a complication of long-term cyclophosphamide use, is uncommon with this short-term therapeutic approach. Spermatogenesis and ovarian function are sometimes adversely affected by the drug, but, as yet, no long-term deleterious reproductive organ effects have been observed, and with short-term therapy, these effects are usually reversible.

Case Illustrating Steroid-Dependent "Nil Lesion" Nephrosis. A 41-year-old man first noted the insidious onset of lower extremity edema in 1968. A renal biopsy was interpreted as either a "nil lesion" or an early membranous glomerulopathy. Therapy with prednisone (40 mg daily) was started and was continued for $4\frac{1}{2}$ months. After 3 weeks, the proteinuria cleared completely, and the dosage of steroids was reduced gradually to 5 mg every other day. Nine months after the initial diagnosis, proteinuria recurred, and prednisone (40 mg daily) plus 6-mercaptopurine was given. The proteinuria again cleared. Two more relapses and remissions occurred with the use of prednisone; however, with each reduction in dose to 30 mg or less, the nephrotic syndrome recurred. The patient was first seen at our institution in August 1970 and had been receiving prednisone therapy (40 mg daily) for 3 weeks. On examination, he appeared to be moderately cushingoid. His blood pressure was 140/110 mm Hg and there was moderate pitting edema in his lower extremities.

There were proteinuria (grade 2) and no urine sediment changes. The level of serum creatinine was 1.1 mg/dl, serum cholesterol 343 mg/dl, and serum albumin 2.56 g/dl. A 24-hr urine protein value was 3.9 g.

Therapy with prednisone was continued for an additional 3 weeks, and with clearing of the proteinuria, cyclophosphamide therapy (150 mg daily) was begun The prednisone dose was gradually reduced and discontinued over 2 months. Cyclophosphamide was then continued for a total of 4 months. Urinalyses during the subsequent 6 years have revealed no recurrence of the proteinuria.

Comment. Repeated courses of steroids or continued use of
moderate steroid dose (20 mg/day) are to be shunned now that
agents such as cyclophosphamide have been shown to be effective in decreasing the rate of relapses. Should a patient experience a relapse shortly after the immunosuppressive program is completed, reassessment of the clinical problem by a
second renal biopsy is advisable.

Cyclophosphamide as the primary agent in "nil disease"
treatment should be a consideration in certain selected cases.[72]
In our experience, it is as effective as steroids when used alone
for 2 to 3 months, a remission occurring usually after 3 to 4
weeks of therapy. Examples of patients who might be candidates for this approach would be those older than 40 years of
age and having some major relative contraindications to the use
of steroids—for example, an active peptic ulcer, previous severe psychotic reaction to steroid use, or severe osteoporosis.

An incomplete (type 3) response or complete lack (type 4)
of response to steroids is an indication for reassessment of the
original diagnosis of "nil lesion" disease. Disagreement among
nephrologists has continued over this particular situation. Some
contend that a complete steroid remission is part of the definition of the "nil lesion" disorder, and if proteinuria persists
with steroid therapy, another disease process is likely to be
present. Others accept these two types of response as compatible with the diagnosis. Until there is more experience with
longer observation and serial renal tissue examinations of these
patients, our knowledge of the clinical spectrum of "nil lesion"
disease will remain incomplete. Practically, if a review of the
renal tissue in this situation does not reveal initially overlooked abnormalities, another biopsy or at least discontinuation of
further steroid use should be strongly considered.

Some lymphoproliferative diseases associated with a nephrotic syndrome have certain characteristics common with
the "nil lesion" nephrotic syndrome.[73,74] More than 75 cases
of lymphoma and nephrosis occurring in close relationship have
been reported. Of interest is the renal lesion that is predominantly seen—indistinguishable from "nil lesion" disease, except for slightly more mesangial hypercellularity. There is no
positive immunofluorescent staining, and electron-dense deposits are not seen on electron microscopy. Most of these patients have had Hodgkin's lymphoma, usually of the nodular
sclerosing type. For reasons not well understood, other lymphoma types more often show renal lesions similar to membranous or mesangiocapillary disease. A definite relationship

between the lymphoproliferative disorder and nephrosis is supported by the response of each disorder to the same therapy. Experience at our institution with nine such patients suggested the following characteristics.[75] The two problems may occur simultaneously, or one may precede or follow the other by a few months. Relapse of the lymphoma is commonly accompanied by reappearance of proteinuria. Treatment of the lymphoma using one of several approaches invariably produces a nephrotic remission. Localized radiation distant from the renal areas or surgical excision of localized lymphoma is equally effective as systemic therapy in treating the nephrotic syndrome. Future study of this type of patient may be productive in identifying the mechanism of glomerular injury in the nephrotic patient with idiopathic "nil lesion." Nephrotic patients with "nil lesion," particularly adults, might be carefully observed for any suggestive clinical signs of an occult lymphoma in view of this relationship.

> Case Illustrating Lymphoma with Nephrotic Syndrome. A 33-year-old man noted the insidious onset of bilateral edema of the lower extremities and a gain in weight during a 3-week period. Six years previously, results of urinalysis had been normal. Physical examination revealed a normotensive male with periorbital and pedal edema.
>
> Laboratory studies showed proteinuria (grade 4) and 6 red blood cells, oval fat bodies, free lipids, and fatty casts per high-power field. The serum creatinine level was 1.2 mg/dl, serum albumin 1.38 g/dl, and 24-hr urine total protein excretion 16.8 g.
>
> Renal biopsy showed only mild mesangial hypercellularity, compatible with a "nil lesion" on light microscopy. Findings on immunofluorescence and electron microscopic studies were unremarkable. The patient was treated with prednisone (60 mg daily) and experienced a spontaneous diuresis in 10 days. Two months later, the 24-hour urine protein excretion was 1.2 g and the serum albumin level was normal. The prednisone dose was gradually reduced and continued at a level of 10 mg daily. At this dosage level, results of repeated urinalyses were normal. However, 22 months later, cervical, inguinal, and axillary adenopathy was noted as well as a return of heavy proteinuria. Biopsy of a lymph node was compatible with Hodgkin's lymphoma. Subsequently, the patient received radiation therapy in 1965, 1967, and 1969 for control of his lymphoma. Proteinuria disappeared. In 1973,

he received nitrogen mustard, vincristine, and prednisone because of lymphoma recurrence. Periodic
follow-up assessment revealed no evidence of recurrent
lymphoma, and results of numerous urinalyses were
negative. The patient died suddenly in 1976 from an
acute myocardial infarction at the age of 45 years.
Autopsy revealed no evidence of Hodgkin's disease.

Comment. The actual incidence of lymphoma developing in association with "nil lesion" nephrosis is very small, but the possibility should be considered during the initial evaluation of any
nephrotic patient with this particular renal lesion. Our understanding of the pathogenesis of "nil lesion" disease may eventually result from an in-depth study of this type of patient. Immunologic techniques available for this unfortunately are still
not sufficiently developed.

Mesangioproliferative Glomerulonephritis

Perhaps 5% of patients with idiopathic nephrotic syndrome have
a morphologic lesion with the following characteristics [76]: (1)
mild, usually generalized (all glomeruli) and focal (some parts
of each glomeruli) mesangial cell increase; (2) scattered mesangial immunofluorescent staining with IgM and complement;
or (3) no distinct electron-dense deposits on electron microscopy.

Nephrologists differ in their assessment of these findings.
Some believe that this is a form of "nil lesion" disease (the
positive findings on immunofluorescence being a nonspecific
mesangial accumulation). A few patients have been reported to
show focal glomerulosclerosis on follow-up biopsy. Others believe that this is neither of the above disorders, but they are
not sure of the group's hemogeneity, considering it a mixture
of several diseases. [77]

In our experience, most of the patients clinically have microhematuria and a few have decreased renal function at the
initial evaluation. [78] Some patients respond to steroids like the
patient with the "nil lesion" nephrotic syndrome does, with
complete resolution of the proteinuria. Most patients, however,
have only a partial response and relapse when the doses of
steroids are reduced. Our success in effecting a sustained remission with the use of cyclophosphamide in several of these
patients has encouraged us to consider this as a possible treatment choice when steroids fail.

Case Illustrating Mesangioproliferative Glomerulonephritis and Possible Renal Hypersensitivity to a Diuretic

A 60-year-old woman was seen in March 1978 with a 2-week history of pedal edema. She had been taking no medications and otherwise felt well. A urinalysis in January 1976 showed no abnormalities. Physical examination at this time revealed a normal blood pressure and moderate pitting edema of both lower extremities. Initial laboratory studies showed proteinuria (grade 4) and 3 red blood cells per high-power field on a routine urinalysis. The serum creatinine level was 1.0 mg/dl, serum albumin was 2.2 g/dl, and a 24-hr urine specimen contained 9.7 g of protein. On light microscopy, renal biopsy revealed focal, mild, segmental mesangial cell increase and no other abnormalities. The immunofluorescent staining revealed IgM, complement, and IgG in the mesangial areas. There were scattered ill-defined electron-dense areas within the mesangium on electron microscopy.

The patient was treated with prednisone 60 mg daily and furosemide. Subsequently, the serum creatinine level increased to 4.0 mg/dl. At this time, furosemide use was stopped because of the concern that a hypersensitivity reaction to the diuretic was occurring. No second renal biopsy was performed, however. The serum creatinine level gradually decreased, and 6 weeks later it was 1.0 mg/dl. At that time, the urinalysis showed proteinuria (grade 2) and a serum albumin level of 3.1 g/dl. Four months later, after the dose of steroids had been reduced, peripheral edema reappeared. The serum protein level at that time was 1.8 g/dl and the 24-hr urine protein quantitation contained 10.0 g. The patient's home physician was advised to begin a course of cyclophosphamide. This recommendation was initially deferred, but later the drug was begun in a dosage of 75 mg/day and continued for 5 months. Follow-up laboratory studies in May 1977 showed that the serum creatinine level was 1.0 mg/dl and that a 24-hr urine specimen contained 270 mg of protein. The cyclophosphamide therapy has since been stopped, and there has been no recurrence of edema formation or heavy proteinuria.

Comment. This patient may have had a form of mesangioproliferative glomerulonephritis. Although the light microscopy findings were compatible with "nil lesion" disease, immunofluorescent staining and electron microscopy findings were equivocal.

There was no clinical evidence of a systemic disease at any time. The patient developed progressive renal insufficiency while receiving furosemide, and with discontinuation of this drug, the renal function returned to normal. During the time that the serum creatinine level was elevated, there was no clinical evidence of vascular volume depletion, so a prerenal component was not considered likely.

Whenever renal insufficiency begins to develop with the use of diuretics, consideration must be given to a hypersensitivity reaction. Frequently, there is no other evidence of this complication, except for the change in renal function. A repeat renal biopsy probably would have revealed either interstitial cellular infiltration or some tubular damage.

With the use of steroids, an incomplete nephrotic remission was noted. However, when the medication was reduced, a full relapse occurred. The subsequent use of cyclophosphamide has resulted in a sustained, complete nephrotic remission.

Focal Glomerulosclerosis

Ten to 15% of the adult population with the idiopathic nephrotic syndrome have focal glomerulosclerosis. With more sophisticated biopsy tissue examination techniques, some patients who are classified as having "nil lesion" disease or focal proliferative disease are now recognized as having focal glomerulosclerosis. It is unclear whether or not this is a single disease entity because similar lesions have been found in patients with asymptomatic proteinuria, and these patients usually do not develop the nephrotic syndrome. Also, the range of clinical conditions associated with this morphologic finding is broad and may encompass other renal disease processes. Lesions indistinguishable from the typical focal sclerosing variety can be seen in association with some types of primary renal disease (such as membranous glomerulonephritis) and also have been described in conditions in which renal damage is possibly due to a mechanical or an infectious cause, such as the chronic renal disease associated with vesicoureteral reflux.[79] The early clinical features of the usual nephrotic patient with this structural lesion appear to be similar to those of the patient with "nil lesion" nephrosis, except for the increased incidence of microhematuria. Later in the clinical course, hypertension appears commonly. Nephrosis sometimes is preceded for months to years by minimal proteinuria. The natural history of focal glomerulosclerosis with the nephrotic syndrome is one of progressive renal function deterioration at a variable rate. In one study, end-stage renal disease was noted in approximately 25% of patients at the end of a 5-year period.[80] Occasionally, spontaneous remissions of the nephrotic syndrome occur. Aside from those patients who have the typical morphologic lesion at the time of initial renal biopsy, the disease should be suspected in any patient who originally was considered to have "nil lesion" nephrosis and who has not responded to steroids.

Debate continues regarding the interrelationship among several renal morphologic groups which include focal glomerulosclerosis, "nil lesion" disease, global sclerosis, and "mesangioproliferative glomerular disease."[81] Much of this confusion emanates from the lack of agreement by renal pathologists and nephrologists as to what constitutes a morphologic and clinical definition of each group. As was discussed earlier, the presence of some mesangioproliferation on light microscopy is considered acceptable by some morphologists in the diagnosis of "nil disease." Also, small amounts of IgM, IgG, and complement in the mesangial region seen on immunofluorescent examination may be acceptable. Some investigators would agree that focal glomerulosclerosis may show this pattern also, and when the specific lesion is not seen on light microscopy or electron microscopy, this should strongly suggest the diagnosis. Others would reject the diagnosis of focal glomerulosclerosis if positive fluorescence is seen in otherwise normal-appearing glomeruli, contending that only the focal lesions show fluorescence with IgM and complement.

Some nephrotic patients have lesions of scattered, completely sclerosed glomeruli unassociated with any other glomerular lesions—so-called global sclerosis. Whether this condition fits into the range mentioned above is also difficult to know. This condition tends to follow a course more similar to "nil lesion" disease than focal glomerulosclerosis, by responding to steroids and infrequently resulting in renal failure.[82]

Perhaps in the early stage of focal glomerulosclerosis or global sclerosis, these lesions, because of their spotty distribution, may be missed, and only with passage of time and observation of the clinical course does the disease process become apparent. This conundrum continues to perplex nephrologists and creates considerable confusion in assessing natural disease courses and responses to various treatment modalities.

Although a very small fraction of patients with focal glomerulosclerosis will respond initially to steroid treatment, relapse is common and is followed by refractory proteinuria.

Most patients, however, show no initial response to either steroids or immunosuppressant drugs. Conservative management directed toward minimizing complications of nephrosis and those associated with the eventual appearance of chronic renal disease is the main objective in following patients who have clearly defined focal glomerulosclerosis.

Case Illustrating Focal Sclerosing Glomerulonephritis
A 36-year-old woman first became aware of swelling in her lower extremities in late 1969. She was initially treated with prednisone, and after 3 weeks a pronounced reduction in weight occurred. The dose of prednisone was reduced gradually to 2.5 mg/day, and the edema recurred in the lower extremities. The dose of prednisone was increased, and at the time of referral the patient was taking 40 mg daily. Examination revealed a normotensive, slightly cushingoid woman with moderate edema of her lower extremities.

Laboratory studies revealed proteinuria (grade 4), free lipids, and oval fat bodies, but no red blood cells. The serum creatinine level was 0.8 mg/dl, serum cholesterol 728 mg/dl, serum albumin 1.63 g/dl, and 24-hr urine protein 6.4 g. Percutaneous renal biopsy was compatible with a "nil lesion." Scattered areas of interstitial fibrosis were seen on light microscopy, and scattered faint areas of IgG were visible on immunofluorescent staining. No electron-dense deposits were noted on electron microscopy.

The dose of prednisone was increased to 60 mg daily and was reduced gradually to 20 mg during a period of $2\frac{1}{2}$ months. The urinary protein excretion decreased to 400 mg/24 hr. With the reduction in prednisone dose to 20 mg, proteinuria recurred. Therapy with prednisone and azathioprine was started. The proteinuria disappeared but recurred 6 months later. At this time, a course of prednisone and cyclophosphamide was given for $2\frac{1}{2}$ months, and again the proteinuria disappeared. The patient continued to check her urine regularly, noting no proteinuria until April 1975, when edema recurred and heavy proteinuria reappeared. She was treated again with prednisone, 60 mg daily, and experienced a complete remission. However, in July, proteinuria gradually appeared and increased in severity. An additional course of prednisone was given in December 1975, with no response. Because of refractoriness to steroids, a second renal biopsy was performed and interpreted as compatible

with focal glomerulosclerosis. The patient has continued to show moderate proteinuria, but unlike most
patients with this lesion and nephrosis, there has been
no biochemical evidence of progressive renal function
deterioration.

Comment. This patient was initially believed to have a "nil lesion" nephrotic syndrome and responded in a compatible man-
ner. Her frequent relapses and eventual steroid resistance
prompted a second renal biopsy, which revealed a focal sclerosing lesion, and no further attempts at treatment were considered. This course is somewhat unusual in that most patients
with this lesion do not experience complete nephrotic remissions or stability of their renal function. A period of time to
observe the clinical course and to obtain additional renal tissue
was necessary before a correct diagnosis was made.

Membranoproliferative Glomerulonephritis

Listed among the primary renal diseases frequently associated
with the nephrotic syndrome, membranoproliferative glomerulonephritis, like others, is predominantly a subclass of the nephrotic syndrome identified by structural renal changes and the
tendency in more than 75% of patients to have a low serum whole
complement or C3 complement level sometime during the
course of the disease.[83] Various morphologic subgroups have
been described (types I, II, and III),[84] but these have contri-
buted little to the choice of therapy and only in a minimal way
to prognosis. Clinically, most (70%) patients present with the
nephrotic syndrome, a few preceded by an upper respiratory
infection and occasionally associated with gross hematuria.
This may lead to some confusion with the diagnosis of acute
poststreptococcal glomerulonephritis, as both diseases are associated with a low level of serum complement. A negative
antistreptolysin O titer in the absence of the recent use of an
antibiotic is helpful in differentiating the two disorders, but the
changes in renal structure are a more definitive finding. The
disorder has been also called "persistent hypocomplementemic
glomerulonephritis and mesangiocapillary glomerulonephritis."
Alternate pathways of complement activation have been demonstrated in the disorder, an observation that will hopefully provide further understanding of immune-mediated glomerular injury mechanisms.[85] Some of the morphologic subgroups have
been associated with the disease "partial lipodystrophy."[86]

The natural history is variable, but progressive deterioration of renal function is common. In some series, the 5-year

survival of the nephrotic patient was less than 50%. Treatment programs using steroids and immunosuppressive drugs have been disappointing and are probably not advisable.[87] Ongoing trials utilizing oral anticoagulant medications and platelet-inhibitor drugs (dipyridamole) are in progress, but the chronic nature and variable natural disease course create major problems in evaluating results of treatment. Treatment trials with these types of drugs, because of their infrequent serious side effects, have been more willingly accepted by clinicians, who must weigh potential advantages against risks of therapy. This is particularly true when, as an alternative, reasonably acceptable approaches to end-stage renal disease will be available to those patients who eventually reach a terminal state.

The remaining primary renal diseases listed in Table 1 (Chap. 1) will not be discussed in detail. Treatment programs for IgG-IgA nephropathy, idiopathic proliferative renal lesions, and rapidly progressive glomerulonephritis have been difficult to interpret, but generally the results are discouraging. IgG-IgA nephropathy is very infrequently associated with the nephrotic syndrome. When they occur together, it portends a poor prognosis.[88] In the few studies reported, no response to any form of treatment has been observed. Some clinicians believe that this disorder may be a form of Schoenlein-Henoch disease because of the renal morphologic similarity, particularly the distinct presence of mesangial IgA staining on immunofluorescence.

Idiopathic proliferative glomerulonephritis likely encompasses many disease processes with variable clinical courses. The generally accepted current approach is one of conservative management, although a short course of high-dose steroid therapy cannot be strongly criticized.

Rapidly progressive glomerulonephritis is, fortunately, an uncommon cause of the nephrotic syndrome. Its clinical course, in the experience of most treatment centers, is one of progressive, usually rapid deterioration of renal function.[89] In view of its recognized poor prognosis, treatment programs using a multidrug approach are often tried; consequently, isolated cases of stabilized or improved renal function cannot be attributed to any single or combination drug program. Some of the patients who do not develop end-stage renal disease have been considered as having poststreptococcal glomerulonephritis, which is self-limited and uninfluenced by any treatment approach.

Approximately 50% of these patients with rapidly progressive glomerulonephritis have an immunofluorescent staining pattern that is indistinguishable from Goodpasture's syndrome (which is considered an antiglomerular basement-membrane-mediated disease).[26] Linear IgG staining is distinct along the capillary basement membrane. Diabetes mellitus and systemic lupus erythematosus also may show this pattern of IgG staining; however, it is never as heavy and distinct as in Goodpasture's syndrome or rapidly progressive glomerulonephritis without pulmonary disease. Whether rapidly progressive glomerulonephritis and Goodpasture's syndrome are variations of the same disease process is unclear. Circulating antibodies to glomerular basement membrane are found in both conditions, however. The clinical course of these two conditions is frequently unrelenting, and end-stage renal disease is a common outcome. Recent attempts at treatment of antiglomerular basement-membrane-mediated disease using plasmapheresis have suggested some encouragement in the management of these patients.[90] The serum levels of antiglomerular basement membrane can be reduced with this procedure, and many institutions have their patients undergo plasmapheresis at the onset once the diagnosis is made. Again, because the disease is variable and other treatment programs are used in conjunction with plasmapheresis, the effect of the technique is difficult to assess. So far, no study has been conducted comparing the results of plasmapheresis alone with those of other commonly used programs, which include corticosteroids and immunosuppressant drugs. (At our institution, several patients receiving only the latter form of treatment have had successful outcomes.) Treatment results probably will need to be evaluated among groups that are comparable in terms of the intensity and duration of the immunologic assault. Presently, this characterization cannot be well quantified by laboratory studies. Exogenous toxic exposure (particularly hydrocarbons) also may be an etiologic factor that contributes an added, almost unmeasurable variable to the treatment assessment of this disease.[91] In summary, Goodpasture's syndrome and rapidly progressive glomerulonephritis are uncommon disorders associated with a high mortality. Patients identified as or suspected of having these conditions should be referred to major medical centers for evaluation and treatment in the hopes that sufficient data will accumulate to determine the efficacy of various treatment programs.

Systemic Diseases Associated with Nephrotic Syndrome

Of the systemic diseases associated with the nephrotic syndrome, diabetes mellitus, sickle cell disease, and Fabry's disease have no recognized effective treatment of the renal involvement. Early treatment observations using platelet-inhibitor drugs in diabetic nephrotic patients possible hold some hope of beneficial effects on proteinuria and renal function stability.[92]

Amyloidosis, either primary or secondary, associated with nephrosis also has no effective form of therapy. A few isolated case reports of the nephrotic syndrome secondary to chronic infection have described the disappearance of heavy proteinuria accompanying eradication of the infection.[93] Ongoing treatment trials of primary amyloidosis using alkylating agents and steroids are in progress, but because of the variable course of both the renal disease and the proteinuria, no predictable drug influence has been demonstrated, at least on the renal deposition of amyloid deposits.

When the nephrotic syndrome is associated with systemic lupus erythematosus, prognosis and treatment programs are frequently dictated by the type of renal structural abnormalities found on renal biopsy. The initial renal lesion, however, may not always continue unchanged, and therefore, considerable difficulty has been encountered by investigators who have attempted to interpret their results of treatment. Three broad categories of lupus renal lesions provide the clinician with general guidelines for therapy.[94]

Systemic lupus erythematosus with a purely membranous lesion similar to idiopathic membranous glomerulopathy often is associated with the nephrotic syndrome. Of interest is the frequently observed, unusually mild extrarenal manifestations of the systemic disease with this lesion. The unfavorable influence of steroids or immunosuppressive drugs (or both) is similar to that seen in idiopathic membranous glomerulopathy, and their use is questionable if only treatment of the lupus renal disease is an indication for these drugs.

Focal proliferative and necrotizing lesions occurring with nephrosis respond more satisfactorily to prednisone therapy (50 to 80 mg/day) given during a minimum of 2 to 3 months, after which the dose is reduced gradually. Whether or not the addition of azathioprine, cyclophosphamide, or chlorambucil is advantageous remains debatable; there is some evidence to indicate that the use of these drugs over a prolonged period is associated with fewer lupus relapses and an improved 5-year survival rate.[95]

The diffuse proliferative renal lesion of systemic lupus erythematosus is uniformly recognized as responding the poorest to any form of treatment. In a few patients, high-dose steroid therapy plus cyclophosphamide may delay the development of progressive renal failure, but aggressive treatment programs often are associated with serious complications related to therapy.

Evidence is accumulating to support a good correlation between the response to therapy of the renal lesion in systemic lupus erythematosus and the improvement of such laboratory parameters as serum whole complement level and anti-DNA levels.[96] Because serial renal biopsy specimens are impractical to obtain, it is hoped that these laboratory tests, in addition to serial renal function measurements, will prove to be reliable guidelines in adjusting the dose of steroids to the lowest level compatible with adequate suppression of renal disease activity. In treating lupus nephritis and the nephrotic syndrome, the continuation of heavy proteinuria is not synonymous with continued disease activity. Once the lupus activity is suppressed, consideration should be given to an alternate-day steroid maintenance program.

The group of vasculitides associated with the nephrotic syndrome is obviously heterogeneous and includes periarteritis nodosa, Wegener's granulomatosis, Schoenlein-Henoch disease, and other entities not readily classifiable. From experience at our institution, the nonclassifiable group in adults has been the most commonly seen. Frequently, these patients are older and have nonspecific symptoms such as fever, malaise, myalgia, and occasional purpuric lesions of the lower extremities. Aside from the nephrotic syndrome and variable degrees of decreased renal function, the commonest laboratory abnormalities are a normocytic hypochromic anemia and a greatly elevated erythrocyte sedimentation rate. High-dose steroid administration often has been effective in halting the inflammatory lesions noted in the kidney glomerulus, but again caution must be exercised in the use of steroids because of the greater intolerance of this medication by older patients. The hemoglobin level, erythrocyte sedimentation rate, and renal function are the most helpful parameters in following the effects of treatment. In most patients, the steroid dose can be reduced from its high level after 4 to 6 weeks. Drug reduction should be followed by frequent clinical assessment, especially when the prednisone dose reaches a level around 20 mg/day. Many of these patients can be weaned from steroids and experience no further flares of their vasculitis.

The efficacy of cyclophosphamide in treatment of this disease constellation appears to be encouraging and awaits further experience. Wegener's granulomatosis, although not usually associated with nephrosis, responds well to this drug. A few reports are equally encouraging for the use of this drug in peri-arteritis nodosa.

Chapter 7

THERAPEUTIC CHOICES FOR END-STAGE RENAL DISEASE

The nephrotic syndrome, with some exceptions discussed previously, often eventuates in end-stage renal disease unless complications from therapy or from the disease itself are fatal. For the primary renal disorders, a major effort in patient management should be directed toward minimizing medical complications that might limit the application of either chronic hemodialysis or renal transplantation. Patients with end-stage renal conditions that are associated with systemic disease present more complex decisions with regard to either of these potential forms of sustaining life.

Chronic hemodialysis is readily available for patients who are not considered candidates for renal transplantation. Although physiologically, emotionally, and logistically it may be a less desirable form of life sustenance, hemodialysis is generally well accepted at present.

When individual patients are evaluated for either of these two procedures, several factors must be considered: (1) the general condition of the patient; (2) the presence of an associated systemic disease that will limit life expectancy; (3) the status of the current systemic disease (quiescent or under control without the use of medication programs that produce major side effects and complications); (4) the availability of access sites for hemodialysis use (a major problem in diabetic patients particularly); (5) the patient's emotional status, which must be stable enough to cope with either of the two types of therapy; (6) the chances of the particular renal disease recurring in a transplanted kidney; and (7) the availability of a suitable living donor or the need for a cadaveric source.

Indications for accepting patients for either of the end-stage treatment programs continue to change, and specific guidelines vary, depending on the philosophy of dialysis-transplant center personnel. Hemodialysis facilities are presently available for most patients with end-stage renal disease. Almost the full cost is now assumed by federal health programs. Perhaps a major unanswered question that faces all dialysis-transplant centers is the quality of life that can be offered to an individual patient by either of these two approaches, when all factors have been considered.

Some general comments regarding end-stage therapy choices for specific renal diseases may be of help to the practitioner who does not deal with these problems continuously. The renal diseases of focal glomerulosclerosis and the dense deposit subgroup of mesangiocapillary glomerulonephritis tend to recur in transplant kidneys with greater frequency than do other primary renal diseases. Recurrence is not always accompanied by reduced renal function, however, and so transplantation continues to be offered to these patients.

Infections related to transplant immunosuppression, chronic transplant rejection, and recurrence of the original disease are the major factors that influence overall prognosis. Patients receiving a renal transplant from a living related donor have a kidney-functioning survival rate according to the National Transplant Registry[97] of 80% for the first year, and this diminishes by 10% per year thereafter. Renal transplantation in patients who have associated systemic disease is more difficult to assess satisfactorily, but one center has reported that the survival rate for those with diabetes is about the same as it is for nondiabetic patients undergoing transplantation.[98] Other centers have not had this experience. Transplantation in diseases such as systemic lupus erythematosus has been reasonably successful, but the numbers of patients involved are small.

Cadaveric transplantation, even with present-day matching techniques, is less satisfactory than transplantation using living related donors. The functioning survival of kidneys for the first year in this group is approximately 50%, and it declines steadily thereafter. Better matching techniques now under study may improve this success rate.

Comparable data for patients who enter chronic hemodialysis programs are difficult to obtain. The patient selection probably presents a bias—older patients and those with major medical problems are not as likely to be accepted for transplantation. Efforts toward improving dialysis techniques continue, but in recent years, no major new methods have been developed that have improved survival. Chronic ambulatory peritoneal dialysis is a more recently available alternative to hemodialysis.[99] A significant limiting factor may be peritonitis and its attendant morbidity. Success of renal transplantation also has remained relatively unchanged since the mid-1970s. A better technique of matching cadaveric donor kidneys with recipients probably is the area in which most progress has been and will be made.

REFERENCES

1. A.G. Kendall, R.C. Lohmann, J.B. Dossetor: Nephrotic
   Syndrome: A Hypercoagulable State. Archives of Internal
   Medicine 127:1021-7, 1971.

2. J.S. Cameron: Histology, Protein Clearances, and Response to Treatment in the Nephrotic Syndrome. British
   Medical Journal 4:352-6, 1968.

3. P. Lim, E. Jacob, L.F. Chio, et al.: Serum Ionized Calcium in Nephrotic Syndrome. Quarterly Journal of Medicine 45:421-6, 1976.

4. S.R. Newmark, C.F. Anderson, J.V. Donadio, Jr., et al.:
   Lipoprotein Profiles in Adult Nephrotics. Mayo Clinic Proceedings 50:359-64, 1975.

5. I.F.C. McKenzie, P.J. Nestel: Studies on the Turnover of
   Triglyceride and Esterified Cholesterol in Subjects with
   the Nephrotic Syndrome. Journal of Clinical Investigation
   47:1685-95, 1968.

6. R.H. Rosenman, M. Friedman, S.O. Byers: The Causal
   Role of Plasma Albumin Deficiency in Experimental Ne-
   phrotic Hyperlipemia and Hypercholesteremia. Journal of
   Clinical Investigation 35:522-32, 1956.

7. D.C. Lowance, J.D. Mullins, J.J. McPhaul, Jr.: Immuno-
   globulin A (IgA) Associated Glomerulonephritis. Kidney
   International 3:167-76, 1973.

8. J.S. Cameron, E.F. Glasgow, C.S. Ogg, et al.: Membranoproliferative Glomerulonephritis and Persistent Hypocomplementaemia. British Medical Journal 4:7-14, 1970.

9. C.G. Becker, E.L. Becker, J.F. Maher, et al.: Nephrotic
   Syndrome after Contact with Mercury: A Report of Five
   Cases, Three after the Use of Ammoniated Mercury Oint-
   ment. Archives of Internal Medicine 110:178-86, 1962.

10. I.A. Jaffe, G. Treser, Y. Suzuki, et al.: Nephropathy Induced by D-Penicillamine. Annals of Internal Medicine 69:549-56, 1968.

11. M.L. Wendland, R.D. Wagoner, K.E. Holley: Renal Failure Associated with Fenoprofen. Mayo Clinic Proceedings 55:103-7, 1980.

12. D.B. Case, S.A. Atlas, J.A. Mouradian, et al.: Proteinuria During Long-term Captopril Therapy. JAMA 244:346-9, 1980.

13. E. Sohar, J. Gafni, M. Pras, et al.: Familial Mediterranean Fever: A Survey of 470 Cases and Review of the Literature. American Journal of Medicine 43:227-53, 1967.

14. R.A. Kyle, E.D. Bayrd: Amyloidosis: Review of 236 Cases. Medicine 54:271-99, 1975.

15. J.H. Felts: Hereditary Nephritis with the Nephrotic Syndrome. Archives of Internal Medicine 125:459-61, 1970.

16. J.-C Brouet, J.-P, Clauvel, F. Danon, et al.: Biologic and Clinical Significance of Cryoglobulins: A Report of 86 Cases. American Journal of Medicine 57:775-88, 1974.

17. R.J.P. Wedgwood, M.H. Klaus: Anaphylactoid Purpura (Schonlein-Henoch Syndrome): A Long-term Follow-up Study with Special Reference to Renal Involvement. Pediatrics 16:196-205, 1955.

18. V. Pardo, J. Strauss, H. Kramer, et al.: Nephropathy Associated with Sickle Cell Anemia: An Autologous Immune Complex Nephritis. II: Clinicopathologic Study of Seven Patients. American Journal of Medicine 59:650-9, 1975.

19. R.A. Gutman, G.E. Striker, B.C. Gilliland, et al.: The Immune Complex Glomerulonephritis of Bacterial Endocarditis. Medicine 51:1-25, 1972.

20. J.A. Diaz-Buxo, R.D. Wagoner, R.R. Hattery, et al.: Actue Renal Failure after Excretory Urography in Diabetic Patients. Annals of Internal Medicine 83:155-8, 1975.

21. Z. Ansari, D.S. Baldwin: Acute Renal Failure Due to Radio-Contrast Agents. Nephron 17:28-40, 1976.

22. J.A. Diaz-Buxo, J.V. Donadio, Jr.: Complication of Percutaneous Renal Biopsy: An Analysis of 1,000 Consecutive Biopsies. Clinical Nephrology 4:223-7, 1975.

23. E.J. Lewis, C.B. Carpenter, P.H. Schur: Serum Complement Component Levels in Human Glomerulonephritis. Annals of Internal Medicine 75:555-60, 1971.

24. W.J. Brzosko, J. Krawczynski, T. Nazarewicz, et al.: Glomerulonephritis Associated with Hepatitis-B Surface Antigen Immune Complexes in Children. Lancet 2:477-81, 1974.

25. C.L. Christian, J.S. Sergent: Vasculitis Syndromes: Clinical and Experimental Models. American Journal of Medicine 61:385-92, 1976.

26. G.J. Beirne, J.P. Wagnild, S.W. Zimmerman, et al.: Idiopathic Crescentic Glomerulonephritis. Medicine 56: 349-81, 1977.

27. C.B. Wilson, F.J. Dixon: Diagnosis of Immunopathologic Renal Disease [editorial]. Kidney International 5:389-401, 1974.

28. F.Llach, A.I. Arieff, S.G. Massry: Renal Vein Thrombosis and Nephrotic Syndrome: A Prospective Study of 36 Adult Patients. Annals of Internal Medicine 83:8-14, 1975.

29. C.S. Winter, R.D. Wagoner, E.J.W. Bowie, et al.: Dysfibrinogenemia and Hypercoagulability in Patients with Membranous Glomerulopathy [abstract]. Thrombosis and Haemostasis 42:67, 1979.

30. M. Goldberg: The Renal Physiology of Diuretics. In Handbook of Physiology. Section 8: Renal Physiology. Edited by J. Orloff, R.W. Berliner, S.R. Geiger. American Physiological Society, Washington, D.C., 1973, pp. 1003-31.

31. E.M. Weyer, H. Hutchins, M.L. McWhiney (eds.): The Physiology of Diuretic Agents. Annals of the New York Academy of Sciences 139:273-539, 1966.

32. F.C. Reubi, P.T. Cottier: Effects of Reduced Glomerular Filtration Rate on Responsiveness to Chlorothiazide and Mercurial Diuretics. Circulation 23:200-10, 1961.

33. C.M. Kagawa, F.M. Sturtevant, C.G. Van Arman: Pharmacology of a New Steroid That Blocks Salt Activity of Aldosterone and Desoxycorticosterone. Journal of Pharmacology and Experimental Therapeutics 126:123-30, 1959.

34. F.C. Reubi: Clinical Use of Furosemide. Annals of the New York Academy of Sciences 139:433-42, 1966.

35. P.J. Cannon, H.O. Heinemann, M.S. Albert, et al.: "Contraction" Alkalosis after Diuresis of Edematous Patients with Ethacrynic Acid. Annals of Internal Medicine 62:979-90, 1965.

36. H. Kjellbo, H. Stakeberg, J. Mellgren: Possibly Thiazide-induced Renal Necrotising Vasculitis. Lancet 1:1034-5, 1965.

37. H. Lyons, V.W. Pinn, S. Cortell, et al.: Allergic Interstitial Nephritis Causing Reversible Renal Failure in Four Patients with Idiopathic Nephrotic Syndrome. New England Journal of Medicine 288:124-8, 1973.

38. A.B. Magil, H.S. Ballon, E.C. Cameron, et al.: Acute Interstitial Nephritis Associated with Thiazide Diuretics: Clinical and Pathologic Observations in Three Cases. American Journal of Medicine 69:939-43, 1980.

39. A.L. Linton, W.F. Clark, A.A. Driedger, et al.: Acute Interstitial Nephritis Due to Drugs: Review of the Literature with a Report of Nine Cases. Annals of Internal Medicine 93:735-41, 1980.

40. H.S. Mitchell, H.J. Rynbergen, L. Anderson, M.V. Dibble: Nutrition in Health and Disease, 16th ed., J.B. Lippincott Company, Philadelphia, 1976.

41. C.F. Anderson, R.A. Nelson, J.D. Margie, et al.: Nutritional Therapy for Adults with Renal Disease. JAMA 223:68-72, 1973.

42. B.T. Burton: Current Concepts of Nutrition and Diet in Diseases of the Kidney. I: General Principles of Dietary Management. II: Dietary Regimen in Specific Kidney Disorders. Journal of the American Dietetic Association 65:623-6; 627-33, 1974.

43. M.M. Avram, H.I. Lipner, A.C. Gan: Medical Nephrectomy: The Use of Metallic Salts for the Control of Massive Proteinuria in the Nephrotic Syndrome. Transactions—American Society for Artificial Internal Organs 22:431-7, 1976.

44. D.A. McCarron, R.J. Rubin, B.A. Barnes, et al.: Therapeutic Bilateral Renal Infarction in End-stage Renal Disease. New England Journal of Medicine 294:652, 1976.

45. W.M. Bennett, G.A. Porter: Efficacy and Safety of Metolazone in Renal Failure and the Nephrotic Syndrome. Journal of Clinical Pharmacology 13:357-64, 1973.

46. H.C. Mitchell, W.A. Pettinger: Long-term Treatment of Refractory Hypertensive Patients with Minoxidil. JAMA 239:2131-8, 1978.

47. A.P. Mukherjee, B.H. Toh, G.L. Chan, et al.: Vascular Complications in Nephrotic Syndrome: Relationship to Steroid Therapy and Accelerated Thromboplastin Generation, British Medical Journal 4:273-6, 1970.

48. J.F. Bridgman, S.M. Rosen, J.M. Thorp: Complications during Clofibrate Treatment of Nephrotic-syndrome Hyperlipoproteinaemia. Lancet 2:506-9, 1972.

49. H. van den Broek, M.T. Han: "Gold Nephrosis." New England Journal of Medicine 274:210-1, 1966.

50. P.A. Bacon, C.R. Tribe, J.C. MacKenzie, et al.: Penicillamine Nephropathy in Rheumatoid Arthritis: A Clinical, Pathological, and Immunological Study. Quarterly Journal of Medicine 45:661-84, 1976.

51. T. Ehrenreich, J. Churg: Pathology of Membranous Nephropathy. Pathology Annual 3:145-86, 1968.

52. D.T. Erwin, J.V. Donadio, Jr., K.E. Holley: The Clinical Course of Idiopathic Membranous Nephropathy. Mayo Clinic Proceedings 48:697-712, 1973.

53. J.S. Cameron: The Natural History of Glomerulonephritis. In Renal Disease, 4th ed. Edited by D.A.K. Black, N.F. Jones. Blackwell Scientific Publications, Oxford, 1979, p. 344.

54. M. Forland, B.H. Spargo: Clinicopathological Correlations in Idiopathic Nephrotic Syndrome with Membranous Nephropathy. Nephron 6:498-525, 1969.

55. W.K. Bolton, N.O. Atuk, B.C. Sturgill, et al.: Therapy of the Idiopathic Nephrotic Syndrome with Alternate Day Steroids. American Journal of Medicine 62:60-70, 1977.

56. Collaborative Study of the Adult Idiopathic Nephrotic Syndrome: A Controlled Study of Short-term Prednisone Treatment in Adults with Membranous Nephropathy. New England Journal of Medicine 301:1301-6, 1979.

57. J.V. Donadio, Jr., K.E. Holley, C.F. Anderson, et al.: Controlled Trial of Cyclophosphamide in Idiopathic Membranous Nephropathy. Kidney International 6:431-9, 1974.

58. J.C. Lee, H. Yamauchi, J. Hopper, Jr.: The Association of Cancer and the Nephrotic Syndrome. Annals of Internal Medicine 64:41-51, 1966.

59. M.G. Lewis, L.W. Loughbridge, T.M. Phillips: Immunological Studies in Nephrotic Syndrome Associated with Extrarenal Malignant Disease. Lancet 2:134-5, 1971.

60. C. Thomson, C.D. Forbes, C.R.M. Prentice, et al.: Changes in Blood Coagulation and Fibrinolysis in the Nephrotic Syndrome. Quarterly Journal of Medicine 43:399-407, 1974.

61. R.D. Wagoner: Unpublished data.

62. F. Llach, S. Papper, S.G. Massry: The Clinical Spectrum of Renal Vein Thrombosis: Acute and Chronic. American Journal of Medicine 69:819-27, 1980.

63. C.V. Harrison, M.D. Milne, R.E. Steiner: Clinical Aspects of Renal Vein Thrombosis. Quarterly Journal of Medicine 25:285-98, 1956.

64. E. Rosenmann, V.E. Pollak, C.L. Pirani: Renal Vein Thrombosis in the Adult: A Clinical and Pathologic Study Based on Renal Biopsies. Medicine 47:269-335, 1968.

65. J. Churg, R. Habib, R.H.R. White: Pathology of the Nephrotic Syndrome in Children: A Report for the International Study of Kidney Disease in Children. Lancet 1:1299-302, 1970.

66. W. Jao, V.E. Pollak, S.H. Norris, et al.: Lipoid Nephrosis: An Approach to the Clinicopathologic Analysis and Dismemberment of Idiopathic Nephrotic Syndrome with Minimal Glomerular Changes. Medicine 52:445-68, 1973.

67. International Study of Kidney Disease in Children: Nephrotic Syndrome in Children: Prediction of Histopathology from Clinical and Laboratory Characteristics at Time of Diagnosis. Kidney International 13:159-65, 1978.

68. V.S. Lim, R. Sibley, B. Spargo: Adult Lipoid Nephrosis: Clinicopathological Correlations. Annals of Internal Medicine 81:314-20, 1974.

69. T.M. Barratt, J.F. Soothill: Controlled Trial of Cyclophosphamide in Steroid-sensitive Relapsing Nephrotic Syndrome of Childhood. Lancet 2:479-82, 1970.

70. J.S. Cameron, C. Chantler, C.S. Ogg, et al.: Long-term Stability of Remission in Nephrotic Syndrome after Treatment with Cyclophosphamide. British Medical Journal 4:7-11, 1974.

71. W.E. Grupe: Chlorambucil in Steroid-dependent Nephrotic Syndrome. Journal of Pediatrics 82:598-606, 1973.

72. A.A. Al-Khader, J.W.K. Lien, G.M. Aber: Cyclophosphamide Alone in the Treatment of Adult Patients with Minimal Change Glomerulonephritis. Clinical Nephrology 11:26-30, 1979.

73. J.M. Kiely, R.D. Wagoner, K.E. Holley: Renal Complications of Lymphoma. Annals of Internal Medicine 71:1159-75, 1969.

74. L. Ghosh, R.C. Muehrcke: The Nephrotic Syndrome: A Prodrome to Lymphoma. Annals of Internal Medicine 72:379-82, 1970.

75. R.D. Wagoner: Unpublished data.

76. A.H. Cohen, W.A. Border, R.J. Glassock: Nephrotic Syndrome with Glomerular Mesangial IgM Deposits. Laboratory Investigation 38:610-9, 1978.

77. W.M. Murphy, A.F. Jukkola, S. Roy, III: Nephrotic Syndrome with Mesangial-cell Proliferation in Children—A Distinct Entity? American Journal of Clinical Pathology 72:42-7, 1979.

78. R.D. Wagoner: Unpublished data.

79. V.E. Torres, J.A. Velosa, K.E. Holley, et al.: The Progression of Vesicourteral Reflux Nephropathy. Annals of Internal Medicine 92:776-84, 1980.

80. J.S. Cameron, D.R. Turner, C.S. Ogg, et al.: The Long-term Prognosis of Patients with Focal Segmental Glomerulosclerosis. Clinical Nephrology 10:213-8, 1978.

81. M. Kashgarian, J.P. Hayslett, N.J. Siegel: Lipoid Nephrosis and Focal Sclerosis: Distinct Entities or Spectrum of Disease [editorial]. Nephron 13:105-8, 1974.

82. R. Habib: Focal Glomerular Sclerosis [editorial]. Kidney International 4:355-61, 1973.

83. R. Habib, C. Kleinknecht, M.C. Gubler, et al.: Idiopathic Membranoproliferative Glomerulonephritis in Children: Report of 105 Cases. Clinical Nephrology 1:194-214, 1973.

84. A.E. Davis, E.E. Schneeberger, W.E. Grupe, et al.: Membranoproliferative Glomerulonephritis (MPGN Type I) and Dense Deposit Disease (DDD) in Children. Clinical Nephrology 9:184-93, 1978.

85. E.H. Vallota, O. Gotze, H.L. Spiegelberg, et al.: A Serum Factor in Chronic Hypocomplementemic Nephritis Distinct from Immunoglobulins and Activating the Alternative Pathway of Complement. Journal of Experimental Medicine 139:1249-61, 1974.

86. D.K. Peters, D.G. Williams, J.A. Charlesworth, et al.: Mesangiocapillary Nephritis, Partial Lipodystrophy, and Hypocomplementaemia. Lancet 2:535-8, 1973.

87. C.D. West: Pathogenesis and Approaches to Therapy of Membranoproliferative Glomerulonephritis [editorial]. Kidney International 9:1-7, 1976.

88. R.C. McCoy, C.R. Abramowsky, C.C. Tisher: IgA Nephropathy. American Journal of Pathology 76:123-44, 1974.

89. K.R. McLeish, M.N. Yum, F.C. Luft: Rapidly Progressive Glomerulonephritis in Adults: Clinical and Histologic Correlations. Clinical Nephrology 10:43-50, 1978.

90. P. Kincaid-Smith, A.J.F. d'Apice: Plasmapheresis in Rapidly Progressive Glomerulonephritis [editorial] . American Journal of Medicine 65:564-6, 1978.

91. G.J. Beirne, J.T. Brennan: Glomerulonephritis Associated with Hydrocarbon Solvents: Mediated by Antiglomerular Basement Membrane Antibody. Archives of Environmental Health 25:365-9, 1972.

92. J.V. Donadio, S.B. Kurtz, J.C. Mitchell, et al.: Platelet Inhibitor Treatment of Diabetic Nephropathy [abstract]. Kidney International 16:915, 1979.

93. J. Lowenstein, G. Gallo: Remission of the Nephrotic Syndrome in Renal Amyloidosis. New England Journal of Medicine 282:128-32, 1970.

94. D.S. Baldwin, J. Lowenstein, N.F. Rothfield, et al.: The Clinical Course of the Proliferative and Membranous Forms of Lupus Nephritis. Annals of Internal Medicine 73:929-42, 1970.

95. J.V. Donadio, Jr., K.E. Holley, R.H. Ferguson, et al.: Treatment of Diffuse Proliferative Lupus Nephritis with Prednisone and Combined Prednisone and Cyclophosphamide. New England Journal of Medicine 299:1151-5, 1978.

96. E.J. Bardana, Jr., R.J. Harbeck, A.A. Hoffman, et al.: The Prognostic and Therapeutic Implications of DNA:Anti-DNA Immune Complexes in Systemic Lupus Erythematosus (SLE). American Journal of Medicine 59:515-22, 1975.

97. Advisory Committee to the Renal Transplant Registry: The 12th Report of the Human Renal Transplant Registry. JAMA 233:787-96, 1975.

98. S.M. Mauer, J. Barbosa, R.L. Vernier, et al.: Development of Diabetic Vascular Lesions in Normal Kidneys Transplanted into Patients with Diabetes Mellitus. New England Journal of Medicine 295:916-20, 1976.

99. D.G. Oreopoulos, M. Robson, B. Faller, et al.: Continuous Ambulatory Peritoneal Dialysis: A New Era in the
Treatment of Chronic Renal Failure. Clinical Nephrology
11:125-8, 1979.

CONTINUING MEDICAL EDUCATION PROGRAM

Medical Examination Publishing Company has joined with Temple University Medical School's Continuing Medical Education Department in establishing a cooperative program for granting CME credit. Temple and MEPC have designed this program to make CME category I credits available to practicing physicians at a reasonable cost. Formal recognition can now be given to the reading a physician does in his home or office of current books in his fields of interest.

This is how the program works. The office for Continuing Medical Education at Temple University School of Medicine has carefully selected appropriate books for Category I CME credits. To obtain credits, the reader must take the post-test, complete the answer sheet according to instructions, and mail to:

> Albert J. Finestone, M.D.
> Associate Dean, Continuing Medical Education
> Office for Continuing Medical Education
> Temple University School of Medicine
> 3400 North Broad Street
> Philadelphia, PA   19140

You should also enclose your check for $10.00 (ten dollars) payable to TEMPLE POSTGRADUATE to help defray administrative costs.

In return, you will receive the correct answers, your graded answer sheet, and, if you have completed the test to the standards of the program, a certificate for the credits you have earned.

The dual objectives of updating your knowledge and securing necessary credits can now be achieved economically. We hope you find this service a valuable and rewarding one.

SELECT THE ONE CORRECT ANSWER FOR QUESTIONS 1-40

1. Thiazide diuretics have their main site of action on renal sodium absorption at the
   A. medullary diluting segment
   B. cortical diluting segment
   C. proximal tubule
   D. distal tubule
   E. none of the above

2. Decreased plasma oncotic pressure in the nephrotic patient initiates the following mechanisms contributing to edema formation, EXCEPT
   A. loss of intravascular fluid into interstitial tissue
   B. stimulation of the renin-angiotensin-aldosterone system
   C. release of antidiuretic hormone
   D. decreased cardiac output
   E. decreased renal blood flow and glomerular filtration

3. The following statements about the dipstick test for urine protein are true EXCEPT
   A. it does not test for Bence Jones protein
   B. grade 4 proteinuria qualitatively represents 1,000 mg/dl
   C. it detects only albumin
   D. grade 3 proteinuria qualitatively represents 300 mg/dl
   E. it is simpler to use than the heat acetic acid method

4. All of the following are major factors influencing serum protein changes in the nephrotic patient EXCEPT
   A. decreased synthesis secondary to dietary alterations
   B. excessive urinary losses
   C. increased catabolism by the renal tubule
   D. the influence of decreased plasma oncotic pressure on protein synthesis
   E. a shift of intravascular proteins into the extravascular compartment

5. The following electrolyte changes are frequently seen in
   untreated nephrotic patients:
   A. Decreased serum calcium
   B. Decreased serum sodium
   C. Decreased serum potassium
   D. Increased serum uric acid
   E. Decreased serum chloride

6. The following drugs are known to cause the nephrotic syn-
   drome EXCEPT
   A. D-penicillamine
   B. mercury
   C. captopril
   D. nonsteroidal anti-inflammatory drugs
   E. tetracycline

7. Purpuric skin lesions in association with the nephrotic syn-
   drome are suggestive of the following diseases EXCEPT
   A. Schoenlein-Henoch disease
   B. a nonspecific vasculitis
   C. focal sclerosing glomerulonephritis
   D. essential mixed cryoglobulinemia
   E. systemic lupus erythematosus

8. Sudden deterioration of renal function in the nephrotic pa-
   tient should suggest the following EXCEPT
   A. contrast media-induced acute renal failure
   B. acute allergic interstitial nephritis secondard to a di-
      uretic agent
   C. acute urate nephropathy
   D. acute renal failure secondary to hypovolemia
   E. acute bilateral renal vein thrombosis

9. A patient with the nephrotic syndrome is found to have light
   chains in his urine and amyloidosis is suspected. In an at-
   tempt to confirm this, the simplest diagnostic procedure to
   be considered next would be
   A. serum whole complement
   B. excretory urography
   C. renal biopsy
   D. electromyogram
   E. rectal biopsy

10. A decreased level of serum whole complement in the ne-
    phrotic patient would be compatible with the following diag-
    noses EXCEPT
    A. idiopathic membranous glomerulopathy
    B. systemic lupus erythematosus
    C. acute poststreptococcal glomerulonephritis
    D. subacute bacterial endocarditis
    E. essential mixed cryoglobulinemia

11. Membranous glomerulopathy in a nephrotic patient may be
    found in all of these conditions EXCEPT
    A. hepatitis B_S antigenemia
    B. systemic lupus erythematosus
    C. Goodpasture's syndrome
    D. D-penicillamine therapy
    E. renal vein thrombosis

12. Which of the following is NOT true? Serum uric acid in the
    nephrotic patient
    A. is best managed with Zyloprim (allopurinol) when lev-
       els greater than 11 mg/dl are found during diuresis
    B. if elevated and associated with hypokalemia is usually
       diuretic drug-related
    C. often is elevated in nephrotic patients with advanced
       renal insufficiency
    D. usually is not associated with gout when elevated in
       patients with chronic renal failure
    E. if elevated, often is associated with uric acid calculi

13. Which of the following electrolyte changes are NOT observ-
    ed during diuresis with loop diuretics?
    A. Hypokalemia
    B. Metabolic alkalosis
    C. Hyperuricemia
    D. Metabolic acidosis
    E. Hyponatremia

14. The following statements about renal transplantation are
    true EXCEPT
    A. it is reasonably successful in patients with systemic
       lupus erythematosus
    B. functioning graft survival rate with caderveric kidneys
       is about 50% for the first year
    C. is more successful with living related allografts than
       with cadaveric kidneys
    D. recurrence of the original disease in the transplanted
       kidney is always accompanied by reduced renal function
    E. is recommended for diabetic end-stage renal disease

15. Which of the following systemic diseases is not associated
    with the nephrotic syndrome?
    A.   Primary amyloidosis
    B.   Diabetes mellitus
    C.   Lupus erythematosus
    D.   Nonspecific vasculitis
    E.   Scleroderma

16. In patients with the nephrotic syndrome and focal glomer-
    ulosclerosis, all of these statements are true EXCEPT
    A.   a very small fraction will respond initially to cortico-
         steroids
    B.   early lesions may be missed because of a spotty dis-
         tribution
    C.   the clinical course is similar to so-called global
         sclerosis
    D.   the morphologic lesion is similar to that sometimes
         seen in vesicoureteral reflux
    E.   it may be difficult to distinguish from "nil lesion"
         disease

17. Which is false? A patient with the nephrotic syndrome and
    "nil lesion" morphology noted on renal biopsy
    A.   rarely develops renal failure
    B.   can be expected to respond to most types of lymphoma
         treatment if the two problems occur together
    C.   should be considered for Imuran (azathioprine) therapy
         if the patient becomes steroid dependent
    D.   infrequently is associated with hypertension
    E.   should be considered for rebiopsy if no response to
         corticosteroids is noted

18. All of these statements concerning percutaneous renal bi-
    opsy are true EXCEPT
    A.   the complication rate is about 7% in large medical cen-
         ters
    B.   most complications can be managed conservatively
    C.   complications are more frequent in patients with mod-
         erately advanced renal insufficiency or hypertension of
         long duration
    D.   biopsy is contraindicated in the solitary kidney
    E.   the fixative solutions for tissue processing in this pro-
         cedure are usually available in any laboratory process-
         ing surgical specimens

19. One of the following is false regarding serum protein ab-
    normalities in the nephrotic syndrome:
    A. The gamma globulin is usually elevated
    B. They are associated with marked edema formation when
        the albumin concentration is less than 1 g/dl
    C. They can be normalized by excessive dietary protein
        intake
    D. They are the major factors responsible for changes in
        the serum calcium
    E. They are of little help in determining the type of renal
        lesion

20. The common maintenance diet recommended for the neph-
    rotic patient consists of all the following EXCEPT
    A. low sodium
    B. low cholesterol
    C. generous amounts of protein
    D. unlimited fluid volume
    E. generous amounts of calories

21. The following statements are true about idiopathic mem-
    branous glomerulopathy and the nephrotic syndrome
    EXCEPT
    A. 50-75% of patients may be expected to reach end-stage
        renal disease in 10 years
    B. spontaneous nephrotic remissions occur in 30-35% of
        cases
    C. immunosuppressive drugs alone or in combination with
        steroids should be avoided in the treatment
    D. the influence of corticosteroids on preservation of re-
        nal function is strongly controversial
    E. it is the most common primary renal disease in adults
        with the nephrotic syndrome

22. Which is true? Serum lipid alterations in the nephrotic syn-
    drome
    A. can be effectively managed with dietary alterations
    B. respond well to the use of clofibrate
    C. have been shown to be responsible for increased vas-
        cular complications in these patients
    D. persist even if the syndrome goes into remission
    E. can be responsible for spuriously low-serum sodium
        levels

23. All of these statements about the nephrotic syndrome as-
    sociated with lymphoma are true EXCEPT
    A. a "nil lesion" morphology is most often associated
       with Hodgkin's lymphoma
    B. heavy proteinuria is caused by renal venous obstruc-
       tion secondary to tumor
    C. relapse of the lymphoma is usually associated with re-
       lapse of the nephrotic syndrome
    D. surgical excision of a localized lymphoma results in a
       nephrotic remission
    E. lymphomas other than Hodgkin's disease often show re-
       nal lesions similar to membranous or membranopro-
       liferative glomerulopathy

24. All of these diuretics are useful in the management of ne-
    phrotic edema EXCEPT
    A. furosemide
    B. acetezolamide
    C. spironolactone
    D. thiazides
    E. ethacrynic acid

25. Which is NOT correct? Furosemide and ethacrynic acid
    A. exert their primary effect on the medullary diluting
       segment
    B. exert their primary effect on the proximal renal tubule
    C. may produce body potassium depletion without effecting
       a diuresis
    D. when given as a bolus will usually increase urine vol-
       ume within 5 min
    E. are more effective diuretic agents than thiazides in the
       presence of renal insufficiency

26. The following statements are true regarding mesangiopro-
    liferative glomerulonephritis and the nephrotic syndrome
    EXCEPT
    A. there is a high incidence of associated malignancy
    B. some patients follow-up biopsy have focal glomerulo-
       sclerosis
    C. most have microhematuria
    D. some nephrologists feel this is a form of "nil lesion"
       disease
    E. may respond to cyclophosphamide when no response to
       corticosteroids is noted

27. Suggested urographic findings of renal vein thrombosis include all of these EXCEPT
    A. enlarged kidneys
    B. decreased concentration of contrast-medium
    C. scalloping of the ureters
    D. elongated and narrowed infundibuli
    E. medially deviated ureters

28. The nephrotic syndrome associated with nonspecific systemic vasculitis has all the following characteristics EXCEPT
    A. normocytic hypochromic anemia
    B. markedly elevated erythrocyte sedimentation rate
    C. fails to respond to corticosteroids
    D. often is accompanied by fever, malaise, and myalgia
    E. sometimes is accompanied by purpuric lesions, particularly of the lower extremities

29. The following laboratory studies are useful in following patients with nonspecific systemic vasculitis and renal involvement EXCEPT
    A. routine urinalysis
    B. erythrocyte sedimentation rate
    C. hemoglobin level
    D. serum creatinine
    E. serum whole complement

30. Clinical features of "nil lesion" nephrotic syndrome include all of these EXCEPT
    A. commonest cause of nephrotic syndrome in pediatric age group
    B. if associated with frequent relapses, cyclophosphamide should be considered
    C. usually associated with moderate renal insufficiency
    D. is rarely associated with red blood cell casts
    E. accounts for 15% of adults with nephrotic syndrome from primary renal disease

31. Factors to be considered at the onset of diuretic attempts in the nephrotic patient include all of these EXCEPT
    A. amount of urine protein
    B. degree of hypoalbuminemia
    C. level of renal function
    D. blood pressure level
    E. history of unstable angina or constant cerebrovascular ischemic attacks

32. Certain obvious states of edema requiring more prompt alleviation include the following EXCEPT
    A. marked pleural effusion
    B. lower extremity edema with skin breakdown
    C. facial edema
    D. separated surgical incision
    E. marked dyspnea from ascites

33. Pulmonary edema in the nephrotic syndrome cannot be explained by
    A. a decreased plasma oncotic pressure
    B. amyloid cardiac infiltration
    C. hypertensive cardiac disease
    D. unsuccessful diuretic attempts with mannitol
    E. unsuccessful diuretic attempts with intravenous serum albumin

34. A common renal disease associated with nephrotic syndrome is
    A. rapidly progressive glomerulonephritis
    B. Goodpasture's syndrome
    C. membranoproliferative glomerulonephritis associated with partial lipodystrophy
    D. Wegener's granulomatosis
    E. Idiopathic membranous glomerulopathy

35. Which of the following diseases would NOT be expected to respond to treatment?
    A. "Nil lesion" nephrotic syndrome
    B. Membranoproliferative hypocomplementemic glomerulonephritis
    C. Nonspecific vasculitis
    D. Wegener's granulomatosis
    E. Nephrotic syndrome associated with Hodgkin's disease

36. Which of the following is NOT true about spironolactone?
    A. It blunts urinary potassium loss due to loop diuretics
    B. It should be used with caution in renal insufficiency because of the risk of hyperkalemia
    C. Gynecomastia is a side effect
    D. Its maximum effect is not reached for 2-3 days
    E. It is the antihypertensive drug of choice in the nephrotic syndrome

37. Which of the following statements is NOT true?
    A. All thiazides appear to act at the same site in the nephron
    B. Hydrochlorothiazide has a duration of action of 24 hr
    C. Short action thiazides are relatively ineffective diuretic agents in the presence of renal insufficiency
    D. Metalazone is effective in a single daily dose regimen
    E. In nephrotic patients with mild edema, thiazides may be used alone for extracellular fluid control

38. The following are components of a routine urinalysis in all nephrotic patients EXCEPT
    A. qualitative proteinuria
    B. free lipids
    C. oval fat bodies
    D. red blood cells
    E. doubly refractile bodies

39. The serum protein electrophoretic pattern in a nephrotic patient has the following characteristics EXCEPT
    A. a monoclonal spike
    B. decreased albumin level
    C. elevated alpha$_2$ globulin level
    D. usually a decreased gamma globulin level
    E. it is similar in most primary renal disorders

40. The following statements about diuretics are true EXCEPT
    A. the most potent are those affecting the medullary diluting segment
    B. proximal tubule acting drugs are relatively ineffective
    C. effectiveness depends to a great extent on the amount of sodium delivered to their site of action
    D. all tend to cause hyperuricemia
    E. furosemide may cause acute hearing loss with intravenous administration

CHOOSE THE FALSE ANSWER FOR QUESTIONS 41-47

41. Causes of unilateral edema of the lower extremities include
    A. deep venous insufficiency
    B. nephrotic syndrome
    C. lymphatic obstruction from malignancy
    D. disparate use of extremities from central nervous system diseases
    E. lymphedema praecox

42. Hypertension in nephrotic patients
    A. may be aggravated by corticosteroid therapy
    B. may not disappear with resolution of the nephrotic
        syndrome
    C. is frequent in nephrotics with poststreptococcal
        glomerulonephritis
    D. is frequent in "nil lesion" nephrotic patients
    E. is managed generally like other forms of hypertension

43. Hypertension in nephrotic patients
    A. is not common during the early course of the renal
        disease
    B. accelerates vascular disease when not controlled
    C. should be controlled even at the expense of some re-
        duction in renal function
    D. is vascular volume dependent
    E. if refractory, should result in consideration of the use
        of minoxidil

44. Dietary alterations in the nephrotic patient
    A. are more effective if diet "control" rather than diet
        "restriction" is emphasized
    B. are best explained late in the patient's hospital course
    C. can be quite palatable when sodium intake is maintain-
        ed at a level of 60-90 meq
    D. are frequently advised but not followed
    E. will be followed better if adjusted to the patient's eat-
        ing habits

45. Urinary free lipids
    A. are indicative of the nephrotic syndrome
    B. may exist as oval fat bodies
    C. may exist as fatty casts
    D. may be mistaken for fats from specimen contamina-
        tion
    E. are doubly refractile because of their cholesterol con-
        tent

46. Attempting to identify the cause for the renal disease in
    newly diagnosed nephritic syndrome is important because
    A. identifying a causitive toxic agent may result in the
        cure
    B. it may uncover an underlying systemic disease
    C. in most instances, it will result in the cure
    D. it aids in assessing renal function prognosis
    E. in adults, a "diagnostic" treatment is unjustified

47. In the treatment of "nil lesion" disease
    A. the steroid-dependent patient should be considered for treatment with cyclophosphamide
    B. a steroid-dependent patient might be considered for treatment with chlorambucil
    C. leukopenic bone marrow suppression is necessary to effect the nephrotic remission
    D. cyclophosphamide treatment of the steroid dependent patient can be expected to produce a 5-year remission in one-half of the cases
    E. a reduction in proteinuria usually occurs within 2-3 weeks after treatment has begun

SELECT THE ONE CORRECT ANSWER FOR QUESTIONS 48-52

48. Which of the following is NOT true about idiopathic membranous glomerular nephropathy with nephrosis?
    A. 15-20% of patients experience a spontaneous remission
    B. 50-75% of patients reach end-stage renal disease in 10 years
    C. The renal lesion may persist despite a nephrotic remission
    D. 50% of patients with this lesion have asymptomatic proteinuria
    E. The renal lesion is indistinguishable from lupus nephritis with membranous changes

49. A nephrotic patient with normal renal function and a serum albumin of 1.0 g/dl is not responding with an adequate diuresis to intravenous furosemide and oral aldactone. The next best step would be
    A. to start intravenous mannitol
    B. to have a thiazide diuretic
    C. to start intravenous albumin
    D. to begin peritoneal dialysis
    E. to put the patient at complete bed rest

50. The following statements about lipid abnormalities in the nephrotic syndrome are true EXCEPT
    A. the most frequent class of abnormality is type II or IIB
    B. there is an inverse relationship to serum albumin level
    C. hypoalbuminemia may be a factor in its genesis
    D. clofibrate is effective in controlling the lipid abnormality
    E. it may be a factor responsible for spuriously low serum sodium levels

51. Choose the false statement regarding aldosterone:
    A. Its synthesis is increased in nephrosis
    B. It influences sodium reabsorption in exchange for potassium in the proximal convoluted tubule
    C. It can be blocked at its nephron site of action by spironolactone
    D. It is increased in nephrotic patients as a result of vascular volume depletion
    E. It has no physiologic shut-off mechanism in the untreated nephrotic patient

52. The following answers are true regarding IgA nephropathy EXCEPT
    A. it is very infrequently associated with nephrotic syndrome
    B. it is responsive to corticosteroid therapy
    C. it may be a variant of Schoenlein-Henoch disease
    D. when associated with nephrotic syndrome, the prognosis is usually poor
    E. it is unresponsive to cyclophosphamide therapy

CHOOSE THE FALSE STATEMENT FOR QUESTIONS 53-100

53. Diagnosis of renal amyloidosis
    A. is made most definitively by electron microscopy
    B. is usually made with the usual light microscopy stains
    C. can be missed unless the pathologist is alerted to the possible diagnosis
    D. should be considered when light chains are found in urine
    E. is most likely present when a patient with multiple myeloma develops a nephrotic syndrome

54. In nephrotic patients sophisticated assessment of renal function with tests such as a creatinine clearance, radioactive I^{125} iothalamate clearance, and insulin clearance
    A. can be misleading
    B. may be subject to error because of low urine flow rates during timed collections
    C. can be helpful in establishing a specific diagnosis
    D. may have a pre-renal variable influence from hypoalbuminemia and vascular volume changes
    E. is not necessary for treatment assessment

55. Coagulation abnormalities in nephrotic patients
    A. revert to normal if there is a nephrotic remission
    B. are no different in patients with and without renal vein
        thrombosis
    C. possibly are a factor in the increased incidence of
        thromboembolic events
    D. should be looked for as a part of the routine nephrotic
        assessment
    E. are not a significant factor in increasing the risks of
        renal biopsy

56. Older nephrotic patients should NOT be diuresed rapidly
    because
    A. of the risk of myocardial damage from hypovolemia
    B. of the risk of cerebrovascular insufficiency from hy-
        povolemia
    C. they cannot tolerate larger diuretic doses compared to
        younger patients
    D. if diabetic, may have an exaggerated tendency towards
        hypotension from diabetic neuropathy
    E. if they have amyloidosis, peripheral neuropathy from
        amyloid deposition will produce an exaggerated ortho-
        static effect

57. Associated clinical conditions which may make diuresis dif-
    ficult in the nephrotic patient include
    A. renal insufficiency
    B. very low serum albumin levels
    C. amyloid cardiomyopathy
    D. lack of dietary cooperation
    E. urinary tract infection

58. Dietary salt substitutes
    A. are well accepted by patients
    B. tend to leave a metallic aftertaste
    C. include lemon juice
    D. must be used with caution in patients taking Aldactone
        (spironolactone)
    E. are generally not necessary in nephrotic patients' pro-
        grams

59. Urinary sodium reabsorption at the distal tubule level
    A. is influenced by the amount of sodium delivered to the
        site
    B. is influenced by the amount of aldosterone available
    C. is influenced directly by thiazides
    D. occurs in exchange for potassium
    E. is increased in the untreated nephrotic patient

60. Intravenous serum albumin
    A.   should be used cautiously in elderly patients with bor-
         derline cardiac status
    B.   should be used aggressively in preparing the nephrotic
         patient for surgery
    C.   is not contraindicated in the presence of renal insuf-
         ficiency
    D.   may precipitate acute pulmonary edema
    E.   is less expensive than mannitol

61. In the management of "nil lesion" nephrosis, the following
    are true:
    A.   The usual treatment initially is prednisone, 60 mg
         q.d. for one month
    B.   Cyclophosphamide is an alternative treatment choice
         when there is a high risk of complications from steroid
         use
    C.   Patients with so-called global sclerosis noted on nee-
         dle biopsy seem to respond differently than those with
         "nil lesion" disease
    D.   A simple way to monitor response is with serial dip-
         stick urine measurements
    E.   Continuation of steroids in steroid-dependent patients
         is not justifiable, as a rule

62. Patients with idiopathic membranoproliferative glomerulo-
    nephritis and the nephrotic syndrome
    A.   may present clinically like patients with acute
         post-streptococcal glomerulonephritis
    B.   have a 90% incidence of low-serum whole-complement
         levels
    C.   do not respond satisfactorily to steroids
    D.   do not respond satisfactorily to immunosuppressant
         drugs
    E.   have been divided morphologically into several sub-
         groups

63. Patients with Goodpasture's syndrome and patients with
    rapidly progressing glomerulonephritis
    A.   should be referred to major medical centers for man-
         agement
    B.   can be recognized morphologically by a granular fluo-
         rescent staining pattern along the capillary wall on re-
         nal biopsy
    C.   have a high incidence of end-stage renal disease
    D.   frequently are found to have serum antibodies to glo-
         merular basement membranes
    E.   have been treated with plasmapheresis with encourag-
         ing results

64. The following statements are true about dieting in nephrotic patients:
    A. Edema control can usually be accomplished after diu-
        resis by using a 120-meq sodium diet
    B. Loss of one pound (0.45 kg) of fat requires the reduc-
        tion of 3,000-3,500 calories
    C. With a 2-g salt diet, a patient receives approximately
        35 meq (1 g) of sodium
    D. Control of dietary sodium in nephrotics is quite pos-
        sible without the use of commercial products low in
        salt
    E. Most foods contain either natural or added sodium

65. Serum calcium levels in nephrotic patients
    A. are low
    B. are influenced by decreased intestinal calcium absorp-
        tion
    C. are influenced by hypoalbuminemia
    D. are often the cause of symptoms
    E. are influenced by the ionized calcium fraction

66. Abnormal serum potassium levels in a nephrotic patients are
    A. almost always diuretic-related
    B. often influenced by the level of renal function
    C. if low and diuretic-induced, correctable by the ad-
        ministration of potassium acetate
    D. may be Aldactone-induced
    E. unrelated to serum albumin levels

67. The following renal diseases causative of the nephrotic syndrome can exist in the absence of the syndrome EXCEPT
    A. membranous glomerulonephropathy
    B. membranoproliferative glomerulonephritis
    C. focal sclerosing glomerulonephritis
    D. diabetic glomerulosclerosis
    E. "nil lesion" disease

68. Pleural effusions in nephrotic patients
    A. are most often bilateral
    B. disappear usually with control of edema
    C. are often a source of significant dyspnea
    D. when associated with pleuritic pain, should raise the
        possibility of a pulmonary embolus
    E. occasionally may require thoracentesis for relief of
        dyspnea

69. Selective proteinuria in the nephrotic patient
    A. is measurable in most clinical laboratories
    B. is characterized by a high percentage of low-molecu-
       lar-weight proteins
    C. often implies a favorable response to steroids
    D. is composed mainly of albumin
    E. is not a practical laboratory test

70. Medications causative of the nephrotic syndrome include
    A. D-penicillamine
    B. mercury
    C. Nalfon (fenoprofen calcium)
    D. gold
    E. allopurinol

71. Infections which have been associated with the nephrotic
    syndrome include
    A. bacterial endocarditis
    B. Haemophilus influenzae
    C. syphilis
    D. ventriculo-atrial shunts
    E. beta-hemolytic streptococcus

72. A nephrotic patient with heavy proteinuria and moderate
    renal failure should be considered for the following:
    A. Bilateral nephrectomy and chronic hemodialysis
    B. Bilateral nephrectomy and transplantation earlier than
       usual
    C. Medical nephrectomy with Gelfoam injection into the
       renal arteries
    D. Further increase in dietary protein
    E. Medical nephrectomy with mercury injection into the
       renal arteries

73. Nephrotic patients with very low serum albumin levels
    A. usually have edema which is not easily controlled
    B. often must accept a greater degree of edema formation
    C. are best managed with periodic intravenous serum al-
       bumin as part of a maintenance program
    D. frequently require the daily use of spironolactone
    E. find a dietary protein intake of greater than 100 g/day
       difficult to achieve

74. Dietary protein of high biologic value includes
    A. cereals   D. fish
    B. eggs   E. meat
    C. milk

75. The basic diet for nephrotic patients with grossly normal
    renal function should consist of
    A. maximum of 1500 ml of water per day
    B. 60-90 meq of sodium per day
    C. maximum high biologic-value protein intake within the
        sodium modification limit
    D. unrestricted potassium intake
    E. unrestricted calcium intake

76. Very high levels of aldosterone production are seen in
    A. the nephrotic syndrome
    B. diabetes insipidus
    C. cirrhosis
    D. a form of adrenal hyperplasia
    E. a form of adrenal tumor

77. The normal glomerular filtrate over 24 hr contains
    A. 144 liters of water
    B. 68 liters of water
    C. 20,000 meq of sodium
    D. 444 g of sodium
    E. some protein

78. During in-hospital-monitored diuresis of a nephrotic
    A. a daily weight record is the best guide for appropriate
        rate of diuresis
    B. uncomfortably edematous patients can safely lose 2-5
        pounds per day
    C. vascular volume adjustments are best monitored by
        supine and upright blood pressure determinations
    D. bed rest is essential
    E. older patients should be more cautiously lowered in
        weight

79. A renal morphologist
    A. should examine renal biopsy tissue by light microscopy,
        immunofluorescence, and electron microscopy techniques
    B. seldom needs clinical information to make a diagnosis
        in the nephrotic patient
    C. must work closely with the clinician involved to arrive
        at a correct diagnosis
    D. should use several additional staining techniques for
        light microscopy when amyloidosis is suspected
    E. functions best when he has access to a continuous and
        generous volume of renal biopsy material

80 A skin rash associated with the nephrotic syndrome
    should suggest the following diagnoses:
    A. Schoenlein-Henoch disease
    B. Systemic lupus erythematosus
    C. Primary mixed cryoglobulinemia
    D. Nonspecific vasculitis
    E. Focal glomerulosclerosis

81. The following statements about mesangioproliferative glo-
    merulonephritis with the nephrotic syndrome are true
    EXCEPT
    A. there is usually IgM noted in mesangial areas on im-
        munofluorescence
    B. this may be a variant of "nil lesion" disease
    C. some patients are found to have focal glomeruloscler-
        osis on follow-up renal biopsy
    D. many patients have either a partial response to ste-
        roids or relapse shortly after steroid doses are tapered
    E. this lesion is seen in approximately 20% of idiopathic
        nephrotic syndrome cases

82. The following statements about the proximal renal tubule
    are true EXCEPT
    A. the greatest percent of sodium reabsorption occurs
        here
    B. it is the site of action of furosemide
    C. sodium reabsorption is accompanied by water reab-
        sorption in this segment
    D. it is the site of action of acetazolamide
    E. Aldactone has no influence on sodium reabsorption in
        this nephron segment

83. The following renal lesions may be associated with gross
    hematuria:
    A. Rapidly progressive glomerulonephritis
    B. IgA nephropathy
    C. Membranoproliferative glomerulonephritis
    D. Acute poststreptococcal glomerulonephritis
    E. Vasculitis

84. Hemoptysis in a nephrotic patient might suggest the follow-
    ing EXCEPT
    A. Goodpasture's syndrome
    B. nonspecific vasculitis
    C. focal glomerulosclerosis
    D. renal vein thrombosis with pulmonary embolus
    E. systemic lupus erythematosus

85. Suggested initial laboratory studies in the evaluation of the
    nephrotic patient might include the following EXCEPT
    A. serum creatinine
    B. serum whole complement
    C. serum protein electrophoresis
    D. SGOT
    E. antinuclear antibody titer

86. Contraindications to percutaneous renal biopsy include the
    following EXCEPT
    A. solitary kidney
    B. allergy to Novocain (procaine hydrochloride)
    C. gross coagulation abnormalities
    D. horseshoe kidney
    E. advanced renal insufficiency with long-standing hyper-
        tension

87. The following statements about hepatitis B antigenemia are
    true EXCEPT
    A. it is not uncommon in membranoproliferative glomeru-
        lonephritis
    B. it is not uncommon in membranous glomerulopathy
    C. it is not uncommon in systemic vasculitis
    D. it does not preclude renal transplantation
    E. it does not preclude chronic hemodialysis

88 In an untreated nephrotic patient, the 24-hr urine specimen
    A. contains less than 10 meq of sodium
    B. contains less than 10 meq of potassium
    C. contains protein mostly in the form of albumin
    D. is less than 100 ml in volume
    E. has a foamy appearance

89. The following statements about systemic lupus erythema-
    tosus with nephritis are true EXCEPT
    A. the diffuse proliferative lesion responds poorly to
        treatment
    B. the best laboratory test to follow in assessing renal
        disease activity is the antinative-DNA level
    C. heavy proteinuria is synonymous with active lupus ne-
        phritis
    D. focal proliferative and necrotizing renal lesions re-
        spond well to steroids
    E. steroid treatment of the membranous lesion is usually
        not effective

90. The following statements regarding "nil lesion" disease
    and the nephrotic syndrome are true EXCEPT
    A. routine urinalysis usually contains red blood cell casts
    B. initially the renal function is usually normal
    C. the response to steroids is usually favorable
    D. it may be associated with lymphoma
    E. it may be misdiagnosed and focal glomerulosclerosis
        missed on renal biopsy

91. The following statements regarding recurrent disease and
    renal allografts are true EXCEPT
    A. focal glomerulosclerosis tends to recur more frequent-
        ly than other primary renal diseases
    B. recurrent renal disease is not always accompanied by
        reduced renal function
    C. proteinuria is a frequent accompaniment of recurrent
        disease
    D. altering the transplant rejection program will influ-
        ence the course of recurrent renal disease
    E. renal biopsy is necessary to establish the presence of
        recurrent disease

92. Among the commonest causes of secondary amyloidosis
    with the nephrotic syndrome are
    A. viral hepatitis
    B. tuberculosis
    C. chronic osteomyelitis
    D. familial Mediterranean fever
    E. parasitic infections

93. The following findings are frequently observed in patients
    with Alport's syndrome:
    A. Microhematuria
    B. Hearing defect
    C. Visual impairment
    D. Orthostatic hypotension
    E. Family history of early deaths from renal disease

94. The distended skin in nephrotic patients
    A. heals slowly from injury
    B. is hypersusceptible to cellulitis
    C. stains positively for IgG and complement on immuno-
        fluorescence
    D. is not unusually sensitive to trauma
    E. is associated with indolent healing and closure separa-
        tion after surgical incisions

95. The nephrotic patient who is edema-free
    A. is usually a young patient with a high protein intake
    B. can use unlimited dietary salt
    C. may be overdiuresed
    D. usually has near-normal levels of serum albumin
    E. may often have orthostatic hypotension

96. The following statements about the four sites of renal tu-
    bular reabsorption of sodium are true EXCEPT
    A. all sites have drugs which can influence sodium reab-
       sorption
    B. the medullary diluting segment is influenced by furo-
       semide
    C. short-acting thiazides affecting the cortical diluting
       segment are effective in the presence of renal insuf-
       ficiency
    D. the proximal tubule accounts for most of the sodium
       reabsorption of the glomerular filtrate
    E. the distal segment exchanges sodium for potassium

97. Treatment for the nephrotic syndrome is effective in the
    following situations EXCEPT
    A. "nil lesion" disease
    B. systemic lupus erythematosus with focal necrotizing
       lesions
    C. Hodgkin's disease
    D. focal glomerulosclerosis
    E. drug-inducednephrosis

98. The following statements about lupus nephritis are true
    EXCEPT
    A. the renal lesion may change during the patient's course
    B. pathologists divide the lesion into three broad catego-
       ries
    C. membranous lupus nephritis morphologically is indis-
       tinguishable from idiopathic membranous glomerulop-
       athy
    D. necrotizing lesions are usually treated for a minimum
       of 3 months
    E. the renal lesion can be predicted from the urinalysis
       characteristics

99. The following statements regarding focal glomeruloscler-
    osis are true EXCEPT
    A. it frequently results in end-stage renal disease
    B. the lesion is seen in reflux nephropathy
    C. the lesion responds to cyclophosphamide
    D. it may occur in the absence of the nephrotic syn-
        drome
    E. it can easily be missed on renal biopsy

100. The following statements about serum albumin in the ne-
    phrotic syndrome are true EXCEPT
    A. the low level can be explained entirely by urinary loss
        of protein
    B. it may improve with an increase in dietary protein in-
        take
    C. usually the lower the serum albumin the more difficult
        the diuresis
    D. it creates a decreased serum oncotic pressure
    E. the level is usually inversely related to the serum
        cholesterol level

ANSWER SHEET

TITLE: The Nephrotic Syndrome: Discussions in Patient Management
by: Richard D. Wagoner, M.D.

INSTRUCTIONS: Blacken the box under the correct answer

	A	B	C	D	E			A	B	C	D	E
1.	☐	☐	☐	☐	☐		40.	☐	☐	☐	☐	☐
2.	☐	☐	☐	☐	☐		41.	☐	☐	☐	☐	☐
3.	☐	☐	☐	☐	☐		42.	☐	☐	☐	☐	☐
4.	☐	☐	☐	☐	☐		43.	☐	☐	☐	☐	☐
5.	☐	☐	☐	☐	☐		44.	☐	☐	☐	☐	☐
6.	☐	☐	☐	☐	☐		45.	☐	☐	☐	☐	☐
7.	☐	☐	☐	☐	☐		46.	☐	☐	☐	☐	☐
8.	☐	☐	☐	☐	☐		47.	☐	☐	☐	☐	☐
9.	☐	☐	☐	☐	☐		48.	☐	☐	☐	☐	☐
10.	☐	☐	☐	☐	☐		49.	☐	☐	☐	☐	☐
11.	☐	☐	☐	☐	☐		50.	☐	☐	☐	☐	☐
12.	☐	☐	☐	☐	☐		51.	☐	☐	☐	☐	☐
13.	☐	☐	☐	☐	☐		52.	☐	☐	☐	☐	☐
14.	☐	☐	☐	☐	☐		53.	☐	☐	☐	☐	☐
15.	☐	☐	☐	☐	☐		54.	☐	☐	☐	☐	☐
16.	☐	☐	☐	☐	☐		55.	☐	☐	☐	☐	☐
17.	☐	☐	☐	☐	☐		56.	☐	☐	☐	☐	☐
18.	☐	☐	☐	☐	☐		57.	☐	☐	☐	☐	☐
19.	☐	☐	☐	☐	☐		58.	☐	☐	☐	☐	☐
20.	☐	☐	☐	☐	☐		59.	☐	☐	☐	☐	☐
21.	☐	☐	☐	☐	☐		60.	☐	☐	☐	☐	☐
22.	☐	☐	☐	☐	☐		61.	☐	☐	☐	☐	☐
23.	☐	☐	☐	☐	☐		62.	☐	☐	☐	☐	☐
24.	☐	☐	☐	☐	☐		63.	☐	☐	☐	☐	☐
25.	☐	☐	☐	☐	☐		64.	☐	☐	☐	☐	☐
26.	☐	☐	☐	☐	☐		65.	☐	☐	☐	☐	☐
27.	☐	☐	☐	☐	☐		66.	☐	☐	☐	☐	☐
28.	☐	☐	☐	☐	☐		67.	☐	☐	☐	☐	☐
29.	☐	☐	☐	☐	☐		68.	☐	☐	☐	☐	☐
30.	☐	☐	☐	☐	☐		69.	☐	☐	☐	☐	☐
31.	☐	☐	☐	☐	☐		70.	☐	☐	☐	☐	☐
32.	☐	☐	☐	☐	☐		71.	☐	☐	☐	☐	☐
33.	☐	☐	☐	☐	☐		72.	☐	☐	☐	☐	☐
34.	☐	☐	☐	☐	☐		73.	☐	☐	☐	☐	☐
35.	☐	☐	☐	☐	☐		74.	☐	☐	☐	☐	☐
36.	☐	☐	☐	☐	☐		75.	☐	☐	☐	☐	☐
37.	☐	☐	☐	☐	☐		76.	☐	☐	☐	☐	☐
39.	☐	☐	☐	☐	☐		77.	☐	☐	☐	☐	☐

	A	B	C	D	E			A	B	C	D	E
78.	☐	☐	☐	☐	☐		90.	☐	☐	☐	☐	☐
79.	☐	☐	☐	☐	☐		91.	☐	☐	☐	☐	☐
80.	☐	☐	☐	☐	☐		92.	☐	☐	☐	☐	☐
81.	☐	☐	☐	☐	☐		93.	☐	☐	☐	☐	☐
82.	☐	☐	☐	☐	☐		94.	☐	☐	☐	☐	☐
83.	☐	☐	☐	☐	☐		95.	☐	☐	☐	☐	☐
84.	☐	☐	☐	☐	☐		96.	☐	☐	☐	☐	☐
85.	☐	☐	☐	☐	☐		97.	☐	☐	☐	☐	☐
86.	☐	☐	☐	☐	☐		98.	☐	☐	☐	☐	☐
87.	☐	☐	☐	☐	☐		99.	☐	☐	☐	☐	☐
88.	☐	☐	☐	☐	☐		100.	☐	☐	☐	☐	☐
89.	☐	☐	☐	☐	☐							

NAME (PRINT) ____

STREET ____

CITY ________________ STATE ________ ZIP __________